"Richard Miller integrates Eastern and Western philosophies for modern trauma therapy. The protocols are written in accessible language to provide tools for professionals, as well as peace of mind for those experiencing PTSD. Miller opens the way for health, healing, and well-being."

—**Mary Ellen Rose**, yoga and meditation instructor at Laurel Ridge Treatment Center, Mission Resiliency Unit, San Antonio, TX

"Richard Miller is an exceptionally skilled practitioner-teacher of both psychotherapy and yoga. His iRest program is a powerful synthesis of both traditions that has proven effective in helping and healing diverse groups of people."

—**Roger Walsh, MD, PhD**, author of *Essential Spirituality*

"Richard Miller's book is the fruit of his lifelong dedication to serve those with PTSD. This book is like having the most loving and compassionate friend with you every step of the way toward complete healing."

—**Swami Dayananda**, integral hatha yoga teacher and trainer, as well as director of LOTUS Center for All Faiths

"Richard's teachings and the practice of iRest offer practitioners the heart of true healing. iRest uncovers the part of you that is untouched by trauma, the part of you that is whole, healthy, and complete—just as it is. I have personally witnessed iRest help thousands of service members, veterans, and military families discover meaning in their traumatic experiences."

—**Molly Birkholm**, cofounder of Warriors at Ease and founder of Healing River Yoga

"Richard Miller's *The iRest Program for Healing PTSD* is an engaging and interactive program for dealing with the underlying issues of PTSD, and not the just the symptoms. Practice and process for healing yourself—what a gift."

—Lee Rodrigues, MA

"What an offering Richard C. Miller has given us! *The iRest Program for Healing PTSD* presents ancient wisdom in an engaging, user-friendly way, and shows how to return to wholeness after being traumatized. This book is the perfect guide to help readers effectively release trauma and recover from PTSD. I highly recommend it."

—**James Baraz**, coauthor of *Awakening Joy* and cofounder of Spirit Rock Meditation Center

"I am grateful for the wisdom of this work and the depth of its practical application. There are useable tools and resources to act as a resilience inoculation to better prepare our military for the challenges they will face, as well as proven and researched practices to assist veterans and their families through the trials and phases of transition from military service. Thank you Richard C. Miller, for your generosity of spirit and for showing us a way forward."

—**John Henry Parker**, behavioral assessment analyst and team development consultant in the field of personal, professional and transformational development, and cofounder of Purple Star Veterans and Families, a non-profit organization providing transition resources to veterans and their immediate and extended family members

"Anyone with a willingness to improve their life can greatly benefit from the powerful pages masterfully written in this book. Richard C. Miller carefully and very clearly lays out a map of tools, techniques, and inner resources that allows us to rediscover the truth of [who] we are; identify and reframe the limiting thoughts, beliefs, and emotions that can keep us stuck; and teach us the self-care skills required to better navigate the obstacles of our journey. "Whether dealing with new life challenges and situations, or the tender scars of old wounds, iRest teaches us to cultivate deeper levels of health, acceptance, awareness, and a greater relationship with ourselves and the world around us. iRest has been instrumental in my own recovery and transition from combat to community, and it is my great hope that through this book, you too will allow Miller to guide you down the path of well-being, to enable you to create a new intention and direction for yourself, and ultimately provide you with the skills and action steps necessary to build your most beautiful life."

> —**Adam McCabe, USMC/OIF 1,OIF 2**, veteran advocate, and founding member and director of the Huts for Vets program in Aspen, CO

"Richard C. Miller articulates with clarity and simplicity an ancient and powerful practice for healing the effects of trauma, insomnia, anxiety, and chronic pain. The practices he presents are easy to follow and integrate into daily living as tools for self-healing. The transformative potential of iRest is made readily accessible through application of the method described so clearly in this book. Having taught this practice to over 2,000 veterans in the Washington, DC Department of Veterans Affairs, I have observed first-hand the potential of iRest in bringing deep rest and relaxation—as well as restoring a sense of well-being and resiliency—into the lives of veterans."

> —**Karen Soltes, LCSW, RYT**, clinical social worker, registered yoga teacher, and certified iRest Yoga Nidra teacher and supervisor

"Precise and profoundly accessible, this book provides the structure and format to skillfully train and compassionately support those trapped in the exhaustive world of repetitive cellular memory known as PTSD. This is an empowering guidebook providing effective techniques that can transform the mechanisms of the brain to create new maps and communication pathways towards enhanced states of physical well-being and peace of mind."

—**Sherri Baptiste**, author of *Yoga with Weights for Dummies* and internationally-recognized yoga teacher and founder of Baptiste Power of Yoga™ and Yoga with Weights: Baptiste Method (www.powerofyoga.com)

"Richard C. Miller provides a breath of fresh air and an easy-to-follow path to help those who struggle with trauma reconnect with their inner peace, wholeness, and joy. His writing is vivid and chock-full with helpful analogies, real-life stories, and transforming practices to show how iRest can heal the wounds of PTSD. I will definitely recommend this book to my college students and the veterans I teach to help them manage stress and experience optimal well-being."

—**Thomas Nassif, PhD**, is a mindfulness researcher and integrative health educator at the Washington, DC Veterans Affairs Medical Center, and serves on the faculty at American University, George Washington University, and Maryland University of Integrative Health

"The well-known and extreme form of stress—PTSD—affects millions of people every day, and can severely impact health and quality of living. So, I was delighted to find this book. Richard C. Miller is not only a trained psychologist, but also a longtime and respected yoga teacher and practitioner. Because of his experience and unique perspective, he offers the latest research and a supportive program to help us all heal and find our inherent joy. I cannot recommend this book highly enough. It is no exaggeration to say it will change your life in wondrous ways."

—**Judith Hanson Lasater, PhD, PT**, author and yoga teacher since 1971

"As both an Operation Iraqi Freedom Army Veteran and a mental health therapist, I know first-hand the struggles that veterans' who suffer from PTSD face. Richard C. Miller has developed an effective, evidence-based protocol which allows veterans to regain control over their emotions and live a more purpose-driven life. I continue to use iRest meditations in both my professional practice, as well as in my private life. Words cannot express the gratitude I feel towards Miller for sharing his work with the brave men and women of US Armed Forces. iRest has empowered thousands of veterans to meet the challenges associated with returning home from combat. I strongly encourage anyone who is suffering from trauma to read this book. It truly does have the power to change your life."

> —Sgt. William Rodriguez, MSW, a decorated three-time Operation Enduring/Iraqi Freedom Combat Veteran who has served three tours of duty in the Middle East as a reconnaissance squad leader with both the 2nd Armored Cavalry Regiment and the 101st Airborne Division (Air Assault)

"Richard C. Miller has distilled a clear, practical, and potent guide to heal PTSD and come home to a deeper sense of yourself. iRest is a wonderful resource!"

> —John J. Prendergast, PhD, psychotherapist, emeritus professor of psychology at the California Institute of Integral Studies in San Francisco, CA, and author of In Touch

The iRest Program for Healing PTSD

A Proven-Effective Approach to Using Yoga Nidra Meditation & Deep Relaxation Techniques to Overcome Trauma

RICHARD C. MILLER, PhD

New Harbinger Publications, Inc.

Publisher's Note

This publication is designed to provide accurate and authoritative information in regard to the subject matter covered. It is sold with the understanding that the publisher is not engaged in rendering psychological, financial, legal, or other professional services. If expert assistance or counseling is needed, the services of a competent professional should be sought.

Distributed in Canada by Raincoast Books

Copyright © 2015 by Richard C. Miller
        New Harbinger Publications, Inc.
        5674 Shattuck Avenue
        Oakland, CA 94609
        www.newharbinger.com

Cover design by Amy Shoup
Acquired by Jess O'Brien
Edited by Marisa Solís

Library of Congress Cataloging-in-Publication Data

Miller, Richard C.
  The iRest program for healing PTSD : a proven-effective approach to using Yoga Nidra meditation and deep relaxation techniques to overcome trauma / Richard C. Miller ; foreword by Eric Schoomaker ; foreword by Audrey Schoomaker.
    pages cm
  Includes bibliographical references.
  ISBN 978-1-62625-024-6 (paperback) -- ISBN 978-1-62625-025-3 (pdf e-book) -- ISBN 978-1-62625-026-0 (epub) 1. Post-traumatic stress disorder--Treatment. 2. Yoga--Therapeutic use. 3. Meditation. I. Title.
  RC552.P67M555 2015
  616.85'2106852--dc23

                                    2014034693

Printed in the United States of America

19   18   17

10   9   8   7   6   5

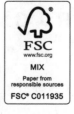

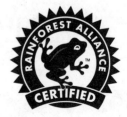

For my loving wife, Anne: I have such deep gratitude for your love, support, and friendship that is always with me every step of my way through this world, as you have also been every step of the way in bringing this book to fruition.

Contents

Foreword

Few challenges to the mind, body, and spirit cause as much widespread suffering and—if untreated—impact the full potential of a human being like that of post-traumatic stress disorder, or PTSD. PTSD is a predictable outcome of natural disasters, such as hurricanes, floods, and tornados, as well as man-made calamities, including violent crimes, war, and terrorist attacks, such as the bombings at Oklahoma City and the Boston Marathon and the 9/11 attacks. It has been a major hurdle in the restoration of service members from all generations and eras in our nation's history. In this insightful book, born of direct personal experience with his own self-care and private practice, and from helping to restore wounded, ill, and injured soldiers and other service members at military and Veterans Administration medical facilities, Richard Miller has provided a classic textbook—a blueprint, really—for teaching people who have experienced trauma not only how to recover but how to thrive!

Richard's approach is laid out simply yet poetically in these pages. He does not offer a quick fix or glib drug-of-the-day choices. Rather, readers will find easy-to-read guidance on the practices of Integrative Restoration, or iRest. Richard shifts the lens on one's view of life and helps us rediscover millennia-old approaches to unlocking the inherent healing power we all possess. With expert guidance, one becomes grounded in the moment, facing off with intrusive thoughts and sensations, using proven methods to effect comprehensive reintegration. iRest made substantial contributions to the recovery of deeply emotionally wounded veterans of a decade of armed conflict at the Walter Reed Army Medical Center in Washington, DC. Richard's work and that of others in the yoga community led the Army Surgeon General's Pain Management Task Force .in 2010 to recommend these practices in the treatment of chronic pain. The following treatise expands that work to PTSD.

Richard offers a "whole person" perspective to sufferers along the entire spectrum of trauma. As providers, our collective mission is to create a safe or sacred space for the traumatized to heal from their pain, no matter what the cause. Richard creates such a space through his comforting guidance without the devastating side effects of medications. This book is a road map with specific directions for traversing the complex, battle-worn road of trauma. It's not just for the suffering soldier but every soul navigating the rocky terrain of this life. For anyone who has ever experienced trauma from which the resulting narrative has held the victim tightly captive, this book is a gift to be cherished. Healing is here for the taking. It is with deep gratitude and humility that Richard offers this gift—the same sentiment that the book elicits in its reader.

—Audrey N. Schoomaker, RN, BSN, E-RYT
Eric B. Schoomaker, MD, PhD, lieutenant
general, US Army (retired)

Acknowledgments

This book would not have been possible without the loving attention, expert guidance, and developmental editing of Jami Macarty. Her understanding with the subject matter and her command of the English language added depth and elegance to my writing. Blessings to you, Jami, for your help and support, and for going beyond the call of duty.

I wish to thank all my teachers, friends, students, and peers who have taught me to bring these precious teachings into the world in a manner that's accessible to all who come to them. To John, for all our years of weekly walks and talks, which have helped shape me and my teachings. To Ross and all my staff, for your loving support throughout this project. To Robin, Karen, and all the iRest teachers, for your dedication to bringing these teachings to veterans and service members everywhere. And to service members and veterans everywhere who have given so much, may the teachings found in this book be of service to you.

Introduction

In 1970, I moved to San Francisco. As a way to meet people in my new city, I signed up for a twelve-week yoga class at the Integral Yoga Institute. As it turned out, the director of the institute decided to have all students be silent in the building during the times I was taking my class. So I didn't meet a single person! I did, however, end up meeting myself; it was a meeting that became a turning point in my life.

At the end of the first practice, the instructor guided the class through a yoga nidra meditation, which involved first deeply relaxing our entire body and mind, and then becoming aware of opposites of sensations, emotions, and thoughts throughout our body and mind, including feeling tense-relaxed, warm-cool, anxious-calm, sad-happy, comfort-discomfort, and upset-peaceful. We were invited to alternate our attention through these pairs of opposites until we were able to embody them with neither aversion nor attachment to what we were experiencing.

I drove home that first evening feeling free of a depression I'd carried within myself for years. I felt expansively present and at ease, radiantly joyful, and deeply connected with myself and everything around me. In that moment, I experienced life as being perfect just as it is. I felt myself to be a spacious, nonlocalized presence at one with the universe around me. Instead of my usual experience of feeling depressed, separate, isolated, and alone, I was having a physical experience of being at peace and connected with both myself and the world around me, unburdened by the thoughts and emotions I'd been carrying around for so long.

While this experience faded over several weeks, it left a longing in me to understand the practice of yoga nidra and to realize myself as this non-separate, peaceful, and connected presence in the midst of my daily life. In the following decades, my yearning would lead me to study with some of the most renowned meditation teachers in the world and to become a skilled practitioner, teacher, scholar, researcher, and pioneer in offering yoga nidra to the world.

How iRest Got Its Name

In 2003, I was invited to consult on a research project at the Deployment Health Clinical Center (DHCC) at Walter Reed Army Medical Center (WRAMC), designed to study the effect of yoga nidra on healing wounded service members experiencing *post-traumatic stress disorder* (PTSD) as a result of their military service. Because *yoga nidra* was an unfamiliar term in military circles and had never been studied as a treatment for PTSD, I was asked to come up with a different name for the particular form of yoga nidra that I teach. I spent months in consultation with my friends, peers, staff, and students trying to come up with a name for this 4,500+-year-old approach to meditation. With their help, I finally decided on the name *Integrative Restoration* (*iRest* for short). I decided on the word *integrative* because this program helps you be a fully functioning, integrated, and healthy human being; I chose *restoration* because it helps you recover joy, peace, and well-being, and it enables you to feel connected to yourself and all of life. The military was delighted with the name. To them, it had a worldly ring that sounded right for a Western-based research study on PTSD.

The study was so successful that iRest was immediately integrated into the DHCC program, where wounded service members were invited to participate in iRest as part of their healing regimen. Based on the success of the WRAMC study, military officials informed me that they were comfortable with my protocol! With respect for the ancient tradition—as well as recognition for a Western name that would be helpful for moving yoga nidra forward in the world of research and in the various military, homeless, university, and other Western-oriented settings I was beginning to bring yoga nidra into—I renamed the program Integrative Restoration—*iRest Yoga Nidra*!

To date, more than twenty successful research studies have been conducted with the iRest program of yoga nidra at VA and military hospitals, and at various universities across North America. More are in the works. Research on iRest is continuing to be conducted with active-duty service members and veterans experiencing PTSD, chronic pain, traumatic brain injury, and sleep disorders, as well as with military hospital health care workers and military couples. The program is also being offered in studies with college students and school counselors experiencing burnout and stress, and with patients undergoing treatment for cancer or multiple sclerosis, as well as with people experiencing substance abuse or homelessness. As a result, iRest is now being taught in military and civilian health and healing settings throughout North America. Trained iRest teachers have also introduced the iRest protocol in Australia, England, Germany, Japan, Iraq, Israel, Palestine, Mexico, Argentina, Venezuela, and other countries around the world.

iRest Is an Open Secret

During my first class in 1970, I discovered a practice that's easy to follow and accessible to everyone who is interested in finding true health, healing, and peace of mind. My own practice—and my work with thousands of men, women, and children during the last forty years—has convinced me that if I, and they, can realize and experience true health, healing, and peace of mind, then so can you. The key to inner peace is not some locked-away secret. It's an "open secret" that's here in plain sight, readily available to you in the pages of this book. And that's why I've written it. I want to put the healing power of yoga nidra in your hands, as a tool you can use to heal your PTSD and trauma, as well as to help you find true health, happiness, and well-being within yourself, in your relationships, and in your daily life—for the rest of your life.

Practice Makes Perfect

You can't know what an apple is unless you taste it. You can't know the power of iRest Yoga Nidra for healing PTSD and trauma unless you practice it. Regular practice of iRest, *a little and often*, enables you to experience the power of the iRest Program for Healing PTSD, as well as achieve optimal health and well-being. This book is designed to help you make iRest your ever-present companion. As you read it, remind yourself: *Little and often...day by day...every day.*

Learning iRest Step-by-Step

After defining PTSD and iRest Yoga Nidra in chapters 1 and 2, this book presents the iRest Program for Healing PTSD step-by-step in chapters 3 through 12. Each of these chapters covers how to weave the ten tools of iRest into your daily life. Each tool builds upon the previous ones and sets the stage for those that follow. As you practice each tool, and then the entire program, you'll grow in your understanding of how and when to use individual tools or the entire protocol to meet your particular needs in any given moment of your life.

Healing unfolds naturally when you apply the tools of iRest throughout your day, each and every day. Allow the tools of iRest to be your trusted resources. They're here to stand by you and to help you respond to every situation, sensation, emotion, thought, and experience you have, throughout all the days of your life.

Instructions for the Guided Practices

iRest Yoga Nidra is, at first, a guided practice. Eventually, you'll be able to practice iRest without a guide or a recording. At first, though, it's helpful to feel the support of a guide. With this in mind, I've created forty-one practice sessions within the chapters of this book. Each is designed to help you learn the iRest program step-by-step, as well as to help you use it in daily life. Each of the forty-one practices in this book has icons ▦ 🔊 that indicate that you should do one or more of the following:

1. Record the practice on your smartphone or computer so that you can listen to the instructions in your own voice.

2. Have a trusted friend read the practice to you. Alternatively, ask your friend to record the practice in his or her voice for you.

3. Download the 42 prerecorded practices to your smartphone or computer and listen to them as audio files. Audio files for eight practices are available for you to stream for free at the iRest website, http://www.iRest.us/practices. The complete set of recordings can be purchased for a fee.

4. Record your answers to questions or reflections to each exercise in a personal journal that you use as you read and engage with the practices in this book.

If you're reading or recording the practice yourself, take time to pause and consider what's being asked of you. Wherever you see three periods (...), pause for several seconds while you consider what the practice is asking of you. If a trusted friend is reading the practice to you, make an agreement with your friend that you will raise your hand as a signal that you'd like to pause before moving on. If you're listening to this meditation as a recording, keep your finger on the pause button so that you can pause and spend time with what's being asked of you before moving on.

It's best to practice iRest in a quiet place, where you can feel secure and at ease, and won't be disturbed by people, animals, or distracting sounds like the ringing of a phone. Find a room where you won't be interrupted. Sit in a comfortable chair or lie down on your bed, couch, or floor. If you're lying down, support your head and neck with a pillow, and place another pillow underneath your knees so that your lower back can relax.

I encourage you to practice iRest in various positions: lying on your back, on your side, or on your stomach; sitting on the floor or on a chair; and while you're standing and even walking around. Eventually, I would like you to practice iRest in every position you find yourself in throughout daily life—bending sideways, twisting, even upside down! This way, when life "twists" you the way it inevitably does, iRest will be at your service. It will be there to help you experience well-being in spite of the position you find yourself in. Ultimately, you'll be able to practice iRest wherever you are, whatever position you're in, under all circumstances.

Moving Forward

As you practice iRest, remember to be gentle with yourself. Healing takes time. Learning iRest takes time. I encourage you to have patience, persistence, and perseverance. You have in your hands a powerful tool for healing your PTSD and for achieving well-being and true peace of mind—wherever you are, whomever you're with, whatever you're doing. I found it.

Others before you with PTSD have found it. Now so have you! Have faith. Have trust. Practice. Then, when the time is right, pay forward what you've learned.

We are all interconnected. Each of us is part of a larger community. It's important to find like-minded people within our community who support us in navigating life successfully. My intention in writing this book is to be part of your community and to pay forward to you the practice of iRest that has been so helpful in my life. I look forward to seeing you in the community and hearing how iRest is serving you. My heartfelt desire is that it leads you to healing, health, well-being, and the interconnected wholeness and peace of mind that are your birthright.

Chapter 1

What Is PTSD?

iRest is the piece that was missing from my PTSD program. It's the one thing I know I'm going to keep doing.

—Vietnam vet

You may be reading this book because you're feeling distress after experiencing or watching a life-threatening event. You may be feeling disconnected and isolated from friends and family, or you may feel that you've lost your interest and joy for life. If you're experiencing any of these symptoms, you may have *post-traumatic stress disorder* (PTSD).

Ted survived multiple explosions in Iraq. Eighteen months after returning stateside, he finds himself feeling afraid and angry over small things that didn't bother him before his tour of duty.

Mary survived a plane crash. Now, one year later, she constantly feels exhausted from waking up in terror at 3 a.m. every night.

Jerry, two years after being robbed at knifepoint, is on constant guard with the feeling that something's always about to go wrong. He's driving around at all times of night, carrying multiple firearms in the trunk of his car "just in case."

Ted, Mary, and Jerry all have symptoms of post-traumatic stress disorder. PTSD describes a pattern of symptoms that have become disabling enough for you to feel limited in your capacity to fully live your life (Kleber, Figley, and Gersons 1995; Wilson, Friedman, and Lindy 2001; Briere and Scott 2006). These are symptoms that emerge as your body and mind attempt to cope with shocking and stressful life events that you've experienced.

You are experiencing PTSD if something distressing has happened in your life and you're having trouble sleeping; finding yourself overly emotional or numb to your emotions; feeling on guard all the time; experiencing painful memories that don't fade; living with a constant sense of fear; or avoiding places, people, or things that remind you of the distressing event. These PTSD symptoms are your body's way of coping with trauma.

What Is a Traumatic Event?

Any event that's life-threatening, causes intense fear, or compromises your physical or emotional safety can cause PTSD. Such events can include the following:

- Suffering a physical injury

- Receiving a serious medical diagnosis

- Being the victim of rape, assault, mugging, or robbery

- Enduring physical, sexual, emotional, or other forms of abuse

- Witnessing or experiencing an automobile, train, or plane crash

- Experiencing or witnessing a natural disaster, war combat, or terrorist attack

- Being the victim of, or being involved in, a kidnapping or torture

- Being involved in a civil conflict

- Experiencing a stressful life event, such as divorce or unemployment, an illness, or the death of a loved one

How Common Is PTSD?

As I write this chapter, there are more than 316 million people living in the United States. An estimated 220 million of us (70 percent) will experience a traumatic event at least once during our lifetime. Forty-four million of us (20 percent) will go on to develop symptoms of PTSD from our experiences. Among US combat veterans, the number of cases of PTSD are even higher. An estimated one in three military combat personnel experiences PTSD. That translates to more than 300,000 veterans from the Middle East war zones alone and 1.7 million veterans from the Vietnam War era experiencing PTSD (Kessler et al. 2005).

While statistics show that most of us will successfully navigate our traumatic life events, heal the various symptoms that are associated with the trauma we experience, and recover our sense of health and well-being, many of us will go on to experience PTSD and need further healing.

What Are the Symptoms of PTSD?

People with PTSD experience key symptoms that can be classified into one of four sets. The first set of symptoms, *arousal*, involves reliving the traumatic event in some way, such as thinking about the event when you're trying to do something else. The second set of symptoms, *numbing*, involves feeling a lack of interest in the things you do or the people you're with. The third set of symptoms, *avoidance*, includes isolating yourself or staying away from places or people that remind you of the traumatic event. The fourth set of symptoms, *vigilance*, involves feeling on guard or startling easily.

Underlying these four basic sets of symptoms are associated issues. People with PTSD may become depressed or develop an anxiety disorder. They may develop dependence on alcohol or drugs. Reckless behaviors, such as excessive gambling and driving at extreme speeds, may be symptoms of PTSD. Gastrointestinal complaints, immune system problems, and other physical illnesses can also have links to PTSD.

Quick Self-Test for PTSD

Read through the symptoms below. Which symptoms are you experiencing? Which symptoms do you believe might be related to a traumatic or stressful event you've experienced? Place a check mark next to those symptoms. Then, below each category, add up the number of boxes you've checked for each set of symptoms.

Arousal

☐ I have trouble falling or staying asleep.

☐ I feel irritable or experience outbursts of anger.

☐ I have troublesome memories, thoughts, or images of the traumatic event.

☐ I have thoughts that frighten me.

☐ There are times when it feels like the traumatic event is happening again.

☐ I experience nightmares or bad dreams.

☐ There are times when I black out or can't remember things.

☐ I have difficulty concentrating.

☐ I have difficulty keeping my attention focused.

☐ I have trouble remembering things that are important to me.

☐ I have difficulty learning new things.

☐ I have physical reactions (e.g., heart pounding, trouble breathing, sweating) when something in my environment (sounds, smells, sights, etc.) reminds me of the traumatic event.

_____ Number of arousal boxes checked

Numbing

- ☐ I feel a lack of interest in activities I used to enjoy.
- ☐ I feel emotionally numb.
- ☐ I seem unable to have loving feelings for those close to me.
- ☐ I feel distant or cut off from other people.
- ☐ I feel emotionally dead inside.
- ☐ I experience feelings of guilt, shame, depression, or worry.
- ☐ I have difficulty making plans for the future.
- ☐ I feel that I won't live as long as I might have before the trauma.

_____ Number of numbing boxes checked

Avoidance

- ☐ I avoid people who remind me of the traumatic event.
- ☐ I avoid places that remind me of the traumatic event.
- ☐ I avoid activities that remind me of the traumatic event.
- ☐ I avoid objects that remind me of the traumatic event.
- ☐ I avoid thinking, talking, or feeling about things that remind me of the traumatic event.

_____ Number of avoidance boxes checked

Vigilance

- ☐ I feel highly alert, watchful, or on guard.
- ☐ I feel jumpy or easily startled by noises, smells, et cetera.

_____ Number of vigilance boxes checked

_____ Total number of symptoms checked from all four categories listed above

_____ Total number of symptoms checked in the categories above that you experience daily

Scoring: Do You Have PTSD?

If you checked a minimum of one symptom that you continually experience daily and five symptoms that cause you distress, and you have been experiencing these symptoms for a minimum of one month, then chances are you're experiencing PTSD (Weathers et al. 1994).

If you suspect that you have PTSD, please consult with a qualified medical doctor or mental health practitioner to get a thorough assessment so that, with his or her help, you can plan a proper course of treatment for yourself. Your course of treatment can include the iRest Program for Healing PTSD that is covered in this book.

Your Nervous System and Trauma

Your nervous system is designed to detect danger and put into action defense mechanisms to ensure your survival as a human being (Porges 2001). Nature has programmed these defense mechanisms in your body to help protect you from overwhelming experiences. These are natural responses to your internal and external life events and stressors. When these mechanisms switch on, they cause you to experience such things as a knot in your belly, tension in your chest, constriction in your throat, pain in your head, and the desire to freeze, fight, or flee. You may also experience a mixture of emotions—including rage, fear, or helplessness—regarding your present, past, or future circumstances. If these stress reactions do not go away on their own, or if they get worse over time, they can overpower your sense of stability and result in your developing PTSD (Porges 2001).

Trauma overactivates your nervous system's mental and emotional circuitry. It leaves you feeling that you're being held hostage by your thoughts and emotions. These thoughts and emotions, in turn, can influence other functions of your nervous system. They can decrease your ability to understand the results of your actions. They can also impair your memory, attention, and concentration. They can get in the way of your healing until long after a trauma-triggering event has occurred (Hebb 1949).

During the past eighteen months, Mark has become paralyzed by fear and anger. He spends most of his days in bed, away from his family and friends. By the time he comes to see me, Mark feels trapped in a spiral of negative thought patterns, unable to move forward with his life.

The "Me" of Trauma

When healing doesn't adequately take place, the same defense mechanisms that are meant to help you survive can instead leave you feeling that something's gone terribly wrong around you and to you. You can also feel that something's now personally and terribly wrong *with* you. In this moment, your *ego* takes over. The ego is the hardwired mechanism within your brain that provides you with a sense of self. It picks up on the feeling that "Something's wrong," then it goes further and affirms, "Something's wrong with me" and "There's something about me that's broken" and "I'll never be the way I was." This happens because your ego identifies with the nonpersonal feeling that "something's wrong." This identification by the ego makes a fact that's not personal—"Something's wrong"—into a very personal self-judgment: "Something's wrong with me." And all this makes difficult what is otherwise a natural process of healing trauma.

How Your Ego Works

It's helpful to understand the function of your personal self, or ego. It is a function that's evolved over millions of years to give you the feeling of being a separate self. Your ego's function is to personalize what are actually nonpersonal events that are just happening in your body and mind (Baumann and Taft 2011). For example, hunger is a body sensation that your ego personalizes by saying, "I'm hungry." Intense sensations in your head are personalized as "I have a headache." Fear that's present as a symptom is personalized as "I'm afraid."

Before eighteen months of age, you had no sense of being a separate self. Back then you just felt sensations of hunger, pain, or fear. This was the same for every taste, sound, sight, sensation, or emotion you experienced. Before this age, you just experienced. You didn't personalize your experience as "mine." Once your ego came online, it began to personalize everything as belonging to "me." That's the ego's job. It personalizes everything. Your ego also does this with whatever arises in your body and mind as a result of your experiencing trauma and symptoms of PTSD. Instead of just feeling strong sensations in your gut or heart, your ego personalizes them as "I'm anxious," "I'm afraid," and "Something's wrong with me."

The family and culture you were raised in also influence how your ego works. As your ego personalizes nonpersonal events, it combines with your personal, family, and cultural values and judgments. These values and judgments can give rise to negative mental and emotional patterns that become lodged in your brain's circuitry. These negative patterns activate cells in your brain, which fire and wire together.

Ted's fear and anger are intensified by his identification with the judgments of people around him, as well as his own negative self-judgments. Instead of saying to himself, These feelings of fear and anger are telling me that something's wrong, he adds fuel to the fire of his fear and anger by constantly judging himself with the belief that having feelings of fear and anger means "Something's wrong with me."

Your Resilient Brain

Research shows that when you experience long-term PTSD, your brain undergoes changes that cause you to experience an increase in negative emotions and thoughts, diminish your concentration and memory, and decrease your ability to understand the results of your actions (Weniger, Lange, and Irle 2009; Bremner 2006; Morey et al. 2012). Fortunately, researchers have also discovered that your brain can change as a result of your life experiences and can reestablish new and healthy connections between your existing brain cells, as well as grow new and healthy brain cells.

As you heal your symptoms of PTSD, your brain grows new and healthy cells. As a result, you gain increased control over your thoughts and emotions. Your concentration and memory increase. Your ability to understand the results of your actions also increases, as does your ability to take productive and positive actions in your life (Lutz et al. 2008; Hutcherson, Seppala, and Gross 2008; Williams et al. 2006; Lemonick 2005; Shin, Rauch, and Pitman 2006).

Treatments for Healing PTSD

All treatments that support the healing of PTSD work by changing your relationship with your traumatic experiences and symptoms of PTSD (Roemer and Orsillo 2003; Tick 2005). Conventional treatments for PTSD include cognitive behavioral therapy, autogenics, progressive muscle relaxation, the relaxation response, eye movement desensitization and reprocessing, and exposure therapy (Najavits 2007; Ready et al. 2006; Foa and Cahill 2002; Saraswati 1998; Miller 2006).

This book offers you another treatment option called *iRest Yoga Nidra*. iRest Yoga Nidra is an ancient meditation-based form of treatment and healing. Like other forms of treatment and healing, iRest works directly by changing the sensory, cognitive, and emotional symptoms that keep your PTSD in place.

Meditation programs, like iRest, are shown to bring about deep relaxation while also producing healthy changes in the structure of your brain, stimulating healing and tissue repair, and providing you self-care skills for changing negative emotions and thoughts into positive ones (Miller 2006). In practical terms, iRest is a meditative practice that enables you to heal the memories, emotions, and beliefs that are signs of your PTSD. iRest provides you with the self-care tools you need to navigate your daily life and restore your inner sense of ease and well-being.

Moving Forward

In the coming chapters of this book I'll offer you written practices, as well as access to online recordings, that support your healing of PTSD. You'll learn the ten tools of iRest Yoga Nidra and how to design your own personal healing practice. You'll also learn how to weave the practices of iRest into your day, so that you can live a healthy and wholesome life. Welcome to the healing practices of iRest Yoga Nidra.

Chapter 2

What Is iRest Yoga Nidra?

iRest Yoga Nidra profoundly changed my life. It turned me right side up as I struggled through treatment for the trauma that had turned my world upside down. My hope is that anyone struggling with his or her own life challenges, or searching for deeper meaning in life, will have the same opportunity to experience the life-giving practice of iRest, as I have.

—T. L., cancer survivor

You can heal your PTSD. As a clinical psychologist and meditation teacher since 1973, I know that it's possible to heal from the symptoms of trauma and PTSD. I've seen the healing take place with my own eyes. The tool I've used to help people heal PTSD and its symptoms is my program, iRest Yoga Nidra, which has helped thousands of people. My program will help you heal your PTSD, too. No matter your background, situation, or circumstance, and no matter how long it's been since your first encounter with trauma or your first symptoms of PTSD, iRest can help you heal your symptoms of trauma, PTSD, and suffering.

The statement "You can heal your PTSD" is a statement of fact. Statements of fact are powerful healing tools, called *intentions*. You'll learn more about discovering and using intentions to aid your healing process as you read on. For now, take a few minutes to positively state these words to yourself: *I can heal my PTSD*. Repeat this declaration to yourself, silently and aloud, several times. As you hear these words, experience the possibility and hope that they spark in your body and mind. Feel the healing power your intentions have. Your intentions, when repeated and asserted as facts, are as important as time, patience, and dedication are to your healing process.

At times your healing process will also involve experiencing negative opposites that arise in response to affirming your positive intentions. In such moments, opposite beliefs such as "Something in me feels so broken that I'll never heal from my PTSD" will arise within you. The iRest Program for Healing PTSD teaches you how to respond to every positive and negative opposite so that your healing of PTSD can be completely successful. For now, affirm and take with you your intention: "I can heal my PTSD."

What Is Yoga Nidra?

Yoga nidra is an ancient meditation practice that supports psychological, physical, and spiritual healing. The term *yoga nidra* is composed of two words from the Indian Sanskrit language:

> *Yoga*: the view, path, and means by which you experience your interconnection with yourself and all of life.

> *Nidra*: changing states of consciousness, such as waking, sleeping, and dreaming, which include sensations, emotions, thoughts, and images.

Yoga nidra is made up of a sequence of meditation practices that help you feel connected to yourself, with others, and to the world around you. These meditation practices teach you how to *respond*, rather than *react*, to your emotions, thoughts, and actions—no matter your state of mind or body. When you *react*, you feel that something remains incomplete in the way you handled a particular situation. Something still feels "off" or "not right." When you *respond*, you feel in harmony with your actions and with the world around you.

What Is Integrative Restoration?

iRest stands for *Integrative Restoration*, which is a modern-day variation of the ancient practice of yoga nidra. iRest Yoga Nidra is a program that teaches self-care skills for healing and resolving symptoms of PTSD. It's an educational practice that focuses on health and healing at all levels of your life: physical, psychological, and spiritual. It's a healing program that respects your age, culture, religion, and philosophical orientation. iRest teaches you self-care tools that lead you to experience self-mastery, resilience, and well-being. iRest Yoga Nidra helps you get back on track, stay on track, heal your PTSD, and get on with living your life with meaning and purpose.

iRest is *integrative*, as it addresses both psychological and physical issues, such as stress, trauma, insomnia, and pain in your body and mind. It helps you feel yourself as a fully functioning, integrated, and healthy human being. And iRest is *restorative* because it helps you recover your inner resources of joy, peace, and well-being, which enable you to feel connected to yourself and all of life. The practice of iRest integrates and restores, so that you can experience well-being wherever you are, whomever you're with, whatever you're doing, and whatever you're experiencing.

Research on iRest

Research reveals the iRest program as a complementary intervention that supports other methods you use to heal your PTSD (Moore et al. 2011). iRest draws upon ancient meditative practices for enhancing well-being and interconnection with yourself and the world around you. And it also incorporates research-proven Western interventions, such as deep relaxation, emotional and psychological healing, and resiliency enhancement.

iRest research participants report a broad range of improvements, including decreases in depression, anxiety, stress, PTSD, chronic and acute pain, and insomnia. They experience greater well-being and serenity, joy, vitality, purpose, and meaning in life. They also report improvements in their interpersonal, marital, and peer relationships, and greater comfort and ability to handle situations they can't control. They experience greater control over their lives and increased ability to handle issues such as PTSD, pain, and stress (Fritts et al. 2014). For a current listing of research using iRest please visit http://www.irest.us/research.

Recommended by the Military

A 2006 research study on iRest, sponsored by the Department of Defense, led the Deployment Health Clinical Center at Walter Reed Army Medical Center to begin providing iRest classes to wounded service members returning from war to help them heal their wartime trauma and PTSD (Engel et al. 2006).

Also based on iRest research, the US Army Surgeon General's Pain Management Task Force listed yoga nidra as a primary approach for pain management in military health care. In addition, the Defense Centers of Excellence (DCoE) have recommended iRest for ongoing research as a treatment for PTSD (Schoomaker 2010; DCoE 2010).

As a result of this and subsequent iRest research and program implementation at the Miami VA; Washington, DC VA; Brooke Army Medical Center; Camp LeJeune; Fort Belvoir; Los Angeles VA; and numerous other military and private facilities, a program is now in place that's bringing group and individual iRest classes to men and women in VA centers, active-duty military facilities, and medical facilities around North America and beyond. Studies at these and other sites join a growing body of research that is taking place at university and clinical settings across North America and abroad.

Tools for Life

I call the various parts that make up the iRest program "tools for life." The iRest program is your tool belt of essential tools to help you heal your symptoms of trauma and PTSD. These tools will empower you to meet each moment of your life, no matter how challenging or difficult, and to achieve unshakable peace and well-being, no matter your circumstance.

This book is designed to help you navigate the complexities of PTSD. I've written it so you can bring these healing tools into your life. These tools will support you to deal with and heal your emotions and thoughts, recover resiliency and joy, and restore meaning, purpose, and value to your life. Since 1973, I've shared these tools with thousands of adults, seniors, and children of all ages, in hospitals and shelters, grade schools and universities, yoga and meditation centers, and military installations and VA centers. After experiencing the program presented in this workbook, those with long-term PTSD said the following:

"iRest helps me experience life—not just live it."

"iRest has given me my first good night's sleep since coming back from war."

"iRest helps me feel in control of my PTSD, instead of feeling that my PTSD is in control of me."

"iRest has taught me to thrive, not just survive."

The Ten Tools of iRest

The ten tools that form the iRest Program for Healing PTSD can be incorporated into every part of your daily life to foster health, healing, and wellness at all levels of your body, mind, and spirit. The chapters of this book are designed to help you understand and practice these ten tools of iRest so that you can heal your PTSD and discover resiliency and well-being in your life and relationships. You'll learn each of the ten tools of iRest in chapters 4 through 12 of this book.

To produce true healing of PTSD, treatment must reach and heal the deepest nooks and crannies within your body and mind. To be effective at that level, the treatment program must be tried and true. The iRest Program for Healing PTSD is such a program. The ten tools of yoga nidra that the iRest program uses have been developed and refined during the past 4,500+ years. These tools have been around for that long because they work! They will transform both your psychological and physical symptoms of PTSD. You may feel that it's not possible to heal and change these symptoms. In fact, the structures within your body and mind are changeable and healable. These ten powerful tools will show you how.

1. Affirming Your Heartfelt Mission

Your *heartfelt mission* is your inner compass of core values that provides purpose and meaning to your life. Discovering and affirming your heartfelt mission helps you get out of bed each morning and keeps you moving forward through your day so that you can attain your life's purpose, no matter what.

2. Affirming Your Intention

Intentions are statements of fact and actions that are guiding forces in your life. Like the banks of a river, intentions keep your life flowing and on course. Intentions are designed to help you heal your PTSD and complete your heartfelt mission.

3. Affirming Your Inner Resource

Your *inner resource* is an inner refuge of constant stability, safety, and well-being. Your inner resource enables you to weather all difficulties you encounter as you heal your PTSD and move through your life.

4. Practicing Bodysensing

Bodysensing helps you experience deep relaxation. It enables you to access information within your body and mind so that you feel grounded and able to respond to every circumstance, no matter how challenging.

5. Practicing Breathsensing

Breathsensing further enhances deep relaxation and well-being through easy-to-learn and easy-to-practice breathing patterns. Breathsensing allows you to connect to the natural healing forces within your body and mind. This connection helps you stay on course and heal your symptoms of PTSD.

6. Welcoming Opposites of Feeling and Emotion

Learning to welcome *opposites of feeling and emotion* teaches you how to respond to negative and positive emotions with actions that empower you and give you a sense of control in your life.

7. Welcoming Opposites of Thought

Learning to welcome *opposites of thought* teaches you how to respond to negative and positive thoughts, images, and memories so that you feel empowered and in control of your life.

8. Welcoming Joy and Well-Being

Joy and *well-being* are your birthright. iRest teaches you how to access the power of joy, well-being, and inner peace in every moment of your life, no matter your circumstance.

9. Experiencing Being Awareness

iRest teaches you how to take a step back and observe your thoughts, emotions, and circumstances from a broader viewpoint so that you can recognize empowering actions that keep you in connection and on course with yourself, others, and your life. Experiencing *being awareness* enables you to understand and experience your wholeness with all of life.

10. Experiencing Your Wholeness

Experiencing your *wholeness* helps you recognize how every situation arrives paired with its perfect response. Recognizing and responding with your perfectly paired response allows you to experience true healing, health, harmony, and well-being in yourself, your relationships, and with all of life.

iRest for the Rest of Your Life

iRest teaches you how to interweave each iRest tool into every relationship and circumstance you encounter, every day of your life, for the rest of your life. iRest teaches you a way of living your life so you can heal your PTSD and feel fully alive and joyful wherever you are, however you are, and no matter who you're with.

Practicing iRest

This book will teach you how to use each tool of iRest as an independent tool, and how to combine some or all of the tools in the way that best suits your needs in any given moment. You may find that what you most often need is Practicing Bodysensing and Breathsensing in order to ease tension, soothe your nervous system, help you get a good night's sleep, or navigate physical or psychological pain, distress, anxiety, or fear. At other times, when experiencing a strong emotion or negative belief or memory, you'll need to use Welcoming Opposites of Feeling and Emotion and Welcoming Opposites of Thought. Sometimes you may need to step away from what you're experiencing to get a moment's rest. Here's where Affirming Your Heartfelt Mission, Affirming Your Intention, Affirming Your Inner Resource, Experiencing Being Awareness, and Experiencing Your Wholeness come in handy. At other times, it will be helpful to take time for Welcoming Joy and Well-Being. Ultimately, integrating these tools of iRest into each moment of your daily life is what the iRest Program for Healing PTSD is all about.

The ten tools of iRest may be likened to foundation stones that you use to build a sturdy house. Each tool enables you to create a strong base for healing your PTSD. Practicing iRest one tool at a time, as several tools together, or as the entire set all at once builds your confidence in the power and effect of these tools. Then, no matter how strong the winds of life blow, you know they can't disturb the house of health and healing that you've built through your practice of iRest.

Core Principles of iRest

The power of the ten tools of iRest rests upon a number of core principles. These core principles are the ground upon which all of the iRest foundational stones sit. The core principles are what make iRest such a powerful program for healing PTSD. Let's take a look at these principles.

Learn to be welcoming.

Stop judging yourself.

Know that everything is a messenger.

Accept what is.

Know that you're always doing your best.

Understand the law of awareness.

Discover your non-separate wholeness.

Practice little and often.

Learn to Be Welcoming

Learning to be welcoming is the core principle that makes iRest such an effective tool for healing PTSD. Welcoming enables you to be *responsive* rather than *reactive*. When you're reactive you're caught in negative patterns that leave you feeling incomplete, out of control, and out of harmony with yourself, others, and life. When you're responsive your actions are authentic, creative, and fresh, leaving you feeling in harmony with yourself. Learning to be welcoming and responsive, rather than refusing and reactive, allows you to gain insight into and control over what's causing your PTSD.

For instance, what would it be like if you arrived at your best friend's home and he or she said, "You're welcome to come in if you'll go away!"? That's not very welcoming. But what if your friend were to say, and truly mean, "You're welcome to come in and stay as long as you need to!"? That would be truly welcoming.

By welcoming each sensation, emotion, thought, person, and situation—just as it is—you grow confident in your ability to respond in ways that "hit the mark." The more you welcome and respond to everything just as it is, in ways that feel right to you, the more confident and empowered you'll feel. The more confident and empowered you feel, the more you'll be able to welcome and respond to all of life's challenges and release long-standing negative patterns of emotions and thoughts. As your capacity to welcome grows, you feel yourself not only welcoming what is, but you also feel yourself *being welcoming*. Being welcoming brings freedom and harmony to your life and actions. Welcoming becomes your state of mind and body.

Stop Judging Yourself

From the point of view of iRest, thoughts, emotions, and actions are classified as either hitting the mark or missing it. With iRest, there's no "good" or "bad" judgments, or "right" or "wrong" ones. When you "miss the mark," you've simply "missed the mark." Similarly, actions that enable you to feel responsive, harmonious, and at peace, where you feel you've "hit the mark," are simply actions where you've "hit the mark." When you hit the mark, you feel in harmony. When you miss the mark, you feel out of harmony.

Negatively judging yourself or others doesn't help anyone. When you judge yourself for being who you are and acting as you do, you end up feeling reactive, contracted, guilty, ashamed, judged, and blamed. You end up telling yourself, *My actions just aren't hitting the mark*, or *I don't feel right inside myself with how I'm responding*, or *My actions feel out of harmony with myself, others, and the world*, or *I feel disconnected from myself, others, and the world around me.*

Negative reactions don't feel good. They also produce further negative reactions. The harmful cycles of guilt, shame, and blame that negative reactions produce prevent you from healing your PTSD. When you're blaming, reacting, and trying to control yourself, others, or life in general, you're trying to get away from experiencing uncomfortable feelings, emotions, or thoughts. But trying to escape or deny these things doesn't work. Fight with reality and you'll always lose. Fighting with yourself doesn't heal; fighting with yourself only increases and keeps PTSD in place. Releasing negative judgments against yourself, and instead welcoming yourself just as you are, is your way through PTSD.

The iRest Program for Healing PTSD teaches you how to stop judging yourself, how to stop reacting in a negative way, and how to take actions that leave you feeling in harmony with yourself and your life in each and every moment.

Know That Everything Is a Messenger

The downside of judging and trying to control yourself or others is that you end up feeling disconnected from yourself, others, and the world around you. The upside of having these feelings is that you can recognize them as *messengers*, or *messages*, that your body's sending to you. These messengers, which can be felt as gut feelings, are asking you to stop, take a breath, feel your body, and get some perspective. From there, you will know what actions you need to take so that you end up thinking, *My actions are hitting the mark*, and *I feel right inside myself and in harmony with how I'm responding*, and *I feel connected to myself, others, and the world around me.*

iRest helps you realize that everything you experience—every sensation, feeling, emotion, and thought—is a messenger that's here to help you stay on track. When you welcome and don't judge yourself, you invite every emotion and thought to come in. You understand that every emotion and thought has a message for you. You know that the sensation, emotion, or thought won't leave until you've fully heard and responded to its message. Your gut feelings, emotions, and thoughts should be considered friends who are here to help heal your PTSD.

Accept What Is

When you judge or try to fix, change, or control your gut feelings, emotions, thoughts, or actions, you're refusing the "what is" of the situation. Welcoming and not judging means you need to first accept the "what is" of a situation. You may not want "what is." You may strongly prefer that things be other than they are. But the "what is" of what you're experiencing *is* what reality is bringing to you in the moment. Remember: when you fight with reality, you always lose.

Stephan was severely depressed when he first sought my help for his PTSD. Thirty years before, while in Vietnam, many of the men he was commanding were killed during a surprise attack while they were out on patrol. Afterward, Stephan suffered a severe mental breakdown, was relieved of duty, and returned stateside for treatment. Underneath Stephan's depression were his deep feelings of guilt, shame, and anger for having survived when men under his command had not.

Our work together consisted of supporting Stephan to stop and welcome his depression, shame, and guilt as messengers that were asking him to go back and look at what had happened that night. This was the beginning of Stephan's journey of accepting rather than trying to escape what had happened. His acceptance of the "what is" of that night took him on a long journey of healing that ended with him sitting down with the other survivors of that ordeal. They were all able to accept that the events of that night had been out of their control. That acceptance led them to find comfort in each other and healing for themselves. In the end, the love Stephan felt for both those who had survived and died replaced his depression. Stephan was finally able to find healing and relief from the burden he'd carried for so many years.

Like it was for Stephan, every feeling, emotion, or thought that you refuse gets pushed into your unconscious mind. Whatever lives in your unconscious ultimately finds its way back into your conscious mind and into your interactions with the outside world. For instance, when you refuse your anger, you'll find yourself in situations that provoke your anger. When you feel guilty, ashamed, or helpless, you'll find yourself in situations that make your guilt, shame, and helplessness rise up. When you judge yourself, you'll feel that others are judging you. Whatever you refuse to deal with comes back around until you learn to welcome it. As you welcome "what is," you begin responding rather than reacting to it. Learning to welcome and respond is part of the process of acceptance. The iRest program teaches you how to accept rather than refuse so that you can feel in harmony and at peace with yourself and the world around you.

Know That You're Always Doing Your Best

You're conditioned by the family and culture you're raised in. You're also conditioned by your socioeconomic status, the food you eat, the millions of years of biological programming you've inherited, and every action you carry out in your life. Just as flowers turn toward light and away from darkness, and animals move toward what's nutritious and away from what's poisonous, you're biologically programmed to move toward pleasure and away from pain. Understanding that you're culturally, personally, and biologically conditioned is a major step in your ability to let go of guilt, shame, and self-judgment—which allows you to heal your PTSD.

The actions you take are neither "right" nor "wrong"; and your actions are not "personal" because they stem from your unconscious cultural, personal, and biological conditioning. Understanding this helps you stop blaming, shaming, and judging yourself. Practicing iRest helps you realize that you're always doing the best you know how. You can set blame, shame, guilt, and self-judgment aside forever when you realize that the way you respond in any given moment is the result of your conditioning up to that moment.

Realizing that you're always doing the best you know how doesn't mean you let go of being responsible for your actions. Rather, realizing that you're always doing your best enables you to take the time to sense your body's internal messengers. Only then can you see the results of your actions. When you see the results of your actions, you gain new information and new conditioning. Your new information and conditioning help you more easily "hit the mark" in the next moment.

Understand the Law of Awareness

Transformation happens easily when you're willing to be aware of and be with "what is." This is what I call the *law of awareness*. Whatever you're willing to place in your awareness, you go beyond. This is because awareness is larger than whatever is within awareness. By feeling yourself as awareness, you're able to gain perspective and see actions you otherwise can't. Awareness is similar to the space around you; it's vast and contains everything. Awareness doesn't refuse anything and isn't attached to anything. It allows everything to be just as it is.

iRest teaches you how to see and rest *in awareness*. From there, you learn how to *be awareness*. Then, you have the capacity to be with anything and everything, no matter how challenging it is. Being aware of your emotions and thoughts allows you to see the larger picture in each and every moment. Experiencing yourself *as awareness* allows you to feel deeply connected to yourself, others, and life.

Discover Your Non-Separate Wholeness

Your five senses and mind work together to perceive the world around you. According to your mind and five senses, the world is made up of separate objects, yourself included. But this isn't the whole story. Actually, as science shows us, everything is a field of energy. If you were to wear special glasses that allow you to see only magnetic fields of energy, you would see how everything blends together as one field of energy. In reality, all objects, including yourself, are non-separate. Everything is energy, which your body experiences as sensation.

▤ ◍ Practice 1: Experiencing Yourself as Sensation

With your eyes open, soften your jaw and allow your shoulders, arms, torso, and legs to relax. Welcome the environment around you as you allow your senses to open to the sounds and perceptions around you.

Notice objects around you as well as your arms, torso, and legs.... Note how your senses and mind, working together, perceive the world around you as made up of separate objects. Note how your body also appears as separate from the objects around you.

Now, close your eyes and sense your body.... Notice how your body is actually a field of sensation that is without a defined border or boundary...a continuation of sensation that extends inwardly and outwardly in all directions.... With your eyes still closed, sense the objects around you.... Notice how they, too, don't have defined borders...how each, in reality, is also a field of sensation.

Now, open your eyes and continue experiencing yourself and the objects around you as fields of sensation. Take your time...just sensing rather than thinking.... Allow the field that is your body to begin to blend with the fields of each object, so that everything blends together as one field of sensation.... Notice how this affects your mind and body....

As you're ready, gently bring movement to your body.... Wiggle your fingers and toes and your arms and legs as you continue to sense your body and the objects around you as a blended and continuous field of sensation.... Feel how this practice affects your state of relaxation as you move back into your wide-awake state of consciousness and go back to reading this book, or move out into the world.

Along with your five senses and mind, you have an additional sense. This sense is designed to perceive your non-separate wholeness with all of life. When your senses and mind work together with this additional sense, you're able to perceive both your unique and separate individuality, as well as your non-separate wholeness with the universe.

When trauma and the symptoms of PTSD put you into survival mode, you instinctively narrow into using only your five senses and mind. You quickly forget your non-separate wholeness. Narrowing down helps you survive. But you need to open up and perceive your non-separate wholeness to fully heal your PTSD. Practicing iRest helps you reexperience your non-separate wholeness with yourself.

Practice Little and Often

The iRest Program for Healing PTSD works best when you consistently practice the ten tools of iRest. Your motto should be *a little and often*. Practicing little and often means as little as a couple of minutes, on a regular basis, each and every day of your life. As you gain skill in iRest, you can engage any of the ten tools in as little as a minute or less. By consistently practicing the ten tools of iRest little and often, you gain trust in their ability to help you respond, heal your PTSD, and thrive in your life and relationships.

Moving Forward

In the following chapters you'll learn how to practice the ten tools of iRest. Keep in mind that while this book introduces these ten tools in order, each tool can be practiced on its own or with others, according to your need in the moment.

Each iRest tool serves a specific purpose. This book helps you learn which tool to use to best address your need in the moment. For example, you can work with Affirming Your Intention or Affirming Your Heartfelt Mission to focus your attention and develop concentration. You can practice bodysensing and breathsensing to relax your muscles and soothe your nerves. You can practice Welcoming Opposites of Feeling and Emotion and Welcoming Opposites of Thought to address specific emotions or thoughts that you're experiencing. You can turn to Affirming Your Inner Resource or to Experiencing Being Awareness and Experiencing Your Wholeness to gain perspective when you're feeling overwhelmed or out of harmony. You see, just as a hammer is for driving nails and a saw is for cutting wood, each iRest tool is designed for a specific purpose. You'll gain maximum benefit as you learn how and when to use each tool.

The iRest Program for Healing PTSD teaches you how to respond to each and every situation, emotion, and thought you experience as you navigate your life, so that you can:

- Experience inner grounding no matter your circumstance

- Experience the core values that provide purpose and meaning to your life

- Depend on your inner resource of safety and security

- Dissolve guilt, blame, and shame

- End self-judgment

- Heal your PTSD

- Restore inner harmony, peace, joy, and well-being in your daily life

- Thrive, not just survive

Healing PTSD is a journey and takes time. Welcome *patience, persistence,* and *perseverance* into your daily routines. Be gentle with yourself. Go slowly. Millions have walked this path. They did it. So can you. With this in mind, take a moment and welcome the following affirmation into yourself:

Just as others have healed their PTSD, I can heal my PTSD.

As you heal, you become a light for those who follow in your footsteps. We are all brothers and sisters on our healing journey together. May you be a light unto yourself, so that those who follow in your footsteps can also affirm:

If he or she healed his or her PTSD, I can heal my PTSD.

Chapter 3

Healing in Wholeness

Instead of feeling that something's wrong with me, iRest helps me feel that there's something right with me.

—Iraq War vet

Traditional therapies are typically designed to address and resolve the symptoms associated with "what's wrong" with you as you undergo treatment for PTSD. "What's wrong" with you is only one side of the coin, or one part of the wholeness reality contains. Continuing to focus only on "what's wrong" can increase the feelings of helplessness and hopelessness related to your trauma. For complete healing to take place, the healing focus has to include the "what's right" side of the coin. iRest is a program that helps you heal "what's wrong" while also enabling you to experience yourself as whole and healthy from the beginning of your healing process. The iRest practices are designed to address both "what's wrong" and "what's right" to resolve your PTSD symptoms so that you can get back on track with your life.

The Difference iRest Makes

From the very first practice, iRest helps you explore and experience within yourself what's already whole and harmonious. This is the part of you that has never been injured and isn't in need of healing. As one soldier said, "I never wanted to face my worst nightmares—my shame, my guilt, my judgments about myself—until iRest showed me that there was a basic goodness about me, that I was okay, in spite of all that I was feeling."

Wholeness is your essential nature. But when you don't recognize and experience your basic wholeness, no matter how much you heal your symptoms of PTSD, you'll always feel that something's amiss. When you realize and feel your wholeness, you recognize within yourself an indestructible resource. This indestructible resource is what allows you to weather the deepest challenges you'll face in life, including the journey to heal your post-traumatic stress.

Healing PTSD takes patience, persistence, and perseverance. It takes time to put into place the necessary internal and external resources that support you to fully address the trauma-inducing events you lived through. By embracing your basic nature of wholeness—which has never been injured or harmed, and doesn't need repair or healing—you'll gain a trustworthy internal friend that will help you heal what has been injured and harmed and what does need repair and healing.

The Power of Being

How do you discover your wholeness? You discover wholeness through experiencing the simple feeling of *being*, which is a universal *felt-sense*, or nonverbal inner knowing, that we all experience (Gendlin 1982). From birth, and throughout every moment of your life, being is a quiet background presence that's always with you but that can go unnoticed until it's directly pointed out. Take a few moments now to feel back through your life and notice how the feeling of being has always been with you. Notice how the feeling of being is something that you directly experience; something that is beyond your ability to describe with words, yet undeniably present and accessible to you, no matter what else you're experiencing.

Experience your felt-sense of being even as you're reading these words, and notice where and how you recognize and experience being in your body. Mindfully experience your felt-sense of being as you read the following words that others have used to describe their felt-sense of being. Do any of their words describe your felt-sense of being?

Indescribable yet undeniable…peaceful…calm…everywhere, yet nowhere specific…warm…heart-centered…presence…loving… safe…connected…refuge…sanctuary…well-being…

Now, take a few moments to pull out your journal and write down words that best describe your own felt-sense of being.

Your Messengers Within

Experiencing being enables you to recognize and experience your wholeness no matter how severe your PTSD. When you forget your felt-sense of being, you can easily lose touch with your non-separate wholeness. Fortunately, when you lose touch with being and your non-separate wholeness, *five special messengers* come in to alert you and help you recover your wholeness. These messengers are natural processes within your body and mind that include your gut feelings, emotions, thoughts, and mental images. They supply you with internal feedback so that you can experience your wholeness as you go about healing your PTSD. Each messenger can arise in either a negative or positive form. Whether negative or positive, each can guide you back to experiencing your essential wholeness and health.

Five Special Messengers

As you forget your wholeness, five internal messengers arise to guide you back home.

Messenger #1		
Limited	versus	**Spacious**
"I feel contracted and limited."		"I feel spacious and whole."

When you forget your basic being, you believe you need more space in order to feel whole again. The solution is to ask yourself, *Where am I when I'm simply being?* Then, experience your basic feeling of being that reveals your *spacious wholeness.*

Messenger #2		
Time-Bound	versus	**Timeless**
"I feel limited by time."		"I feel timeless and whole."

When you forget your basic being, you believe you need more time in order to feel whole again. The solution is to ask yourself, *When am I when I'm simply being?* Then experience your basic feeling of being that reveals your *timeless wholeness.*

Messenger #3		
Lacking and Flawed	versus	**Perfect**
"I feel that I'm lacking and flawed."		"I feel perfect and whole."

When you forget your basic being, you believe you're lacking and need to acquire something in order to feel whole again. The solution is to ask yourself, *How am I when I'm simply being?* Then experience your basic feeling of being that reveals your *perfect wholeness.*

Messenger #4		
Disconnected	versus	**Connected**
"I feel confused and disconnected."		"I feel connected and whole."

When you forget your basic being, you feel confused and disconnected. You believe there's something you must understand in order to feel whole again. The solution is to ask yourself, *What am I when I'm simply being?* Then experience your basic feeling of being that reveals your *connected wholeness.*

Messenger #5		
Incomplete	versus	**Complete**
"I feel incomplete."		"I feel whole."

When you forget your basic being, you believe there's something you need to do in order to feel complete and whole again. The solution is to ask yourself, *Who am I when I'm simply being?* Then experience your basic feeling of being that reveals your *complete wholeness.*

These five messengers are feelings that you experience within your body. They are the product of your genetic inheritance from millions of years of bioengineering. Nature has wired these messengers into your nervous system so that you can experience yourself as both a separate individual and as the non-separate wholeness of life. These messengers are designed to help you recognize that every sensation, emotion, and thought you experience—every fear, anxiety, anger, hurt, shame, depression, joy, or delight that you feel—is a messenger that can directly reveal your deepest psychological and spiritual health, harmony, and wholeness of being.

Experiencing Being and Wholeness with Your Five Special Messengers

The following practice is designed to reacquaint you with your basic being as the doorway that leads to your experiencing your basic wholeness, health, and well-being. Your ability to access being and wholeness at a moment's notice provides you with an ever-present tool that you can use to heal your PTSD. As you move through this practice, take as much time as you need with each section before moving on to the next part.

Practice 2: Messenger Meditation

Lie or sit in a comfortable position. Open your senses to your surroundings: sound...color...light.... Open to the feeling of the environment around you... the touch of air on your skin...the sensations where your body touches the surface that's providing support...the feeling of your entire body...and your felt-sense of simply being.... Take a moment and enjoy this moment of simply being.... Take delight in not having to be somewhere.... Let go of what-ever you were previously doing or thinking.... Just being...nothing to do... nowhere to go.... Simply enjoy the easy feeling of just being.... Merge with and lose your sense of separation from this feeling of being.... Feel yourself not just *in* being but completely absorbed *as* being.... Become being....

As you listen to each of the following questions, let go of everything you've previously heard or experienced.... Enjoy the easy feeling of simply being while you answer each question from your own experience as being....

1st Messenger. Feeling and experiencing yourself as being, when you're just being, how would you describe your experience of where you're located in space?... Where, for instance is your innermost center and outermost boundary?... When you're just being, do you have a distinct border or boundary?...

2nd Messenger. When you're just being, without going into thinking or memory, what's your experience of time?...

3rd Messenger. When you're just being, is there anything that you need to acquire that will make you any better or more perfect than you already are as being?...

4th Messenger. When you're just being, is there anything you need to understand that would make you any more connected than you already are as being?...

5th Messenger. When you're just being, is there anything you need to do that, by accomplishing it, would make you any more complete than you already are as being?...

Take a few moments now to simply be...without going into memory or thinking.... Feel your wholeness of being...spacious...timeless...perfect... connected...complete...just as you are...just as it is...without going into thinking...just being....

As you're ready...taking your time...while experiencing the feeling of being and wholeness...sense your physical body...and the feeling of being.... Feel the sensation of your body touching the surface that's supporting it... and the feeling of being...the touch of air on your skin...and the feeling of being...light, color, and sound...and the feeling of being...the feeling of the space around you...and the feeling of being....

Now, open your eyes and notice what you see, hear, and feel...while also noticing the feeling of being.... Now close your eyes and reaffirm the feeling of being.... Now open and close your eyes several times while continuing to affirm the feeling of being....

Now, as you're ready, come back to sensing yourself fully alert, with your eyes open, feeling present to this moment...your body...your thoughts...your emotions...the environment around you...even as you continue to experience your underlying feeling of being and wholeness....

Experiencing your felt-sense of being and wholeness in your daily life has a powerful effect on healing your PTSD. Let's look at those effects now.

Messenger #1: Contracted and Limited Versus Spacious and Whole

"When you're simply being, how would you describe your felt-sense of location? Where are you when you're simply being?" When I posed these two questions during an iRest class at a homeless shelter, one woman responded, "As being, I feel myself as an indescribable presence that's everywhere and nowhere in particular."

In your journal, write down words that best describe your felt-sense of location when you're just being.

You can't deny the feeling of being. But being doesn't have a distinct location with a defined center or boundary. It's a boundless field of presence. It's everywhere and nowhere specific. So, one description of yourself as being is that you are *an undeniable presence that's spacious, unlimited, and whole.*

Messenger #2: Time-Bound Versus Timeless

When you're simply being, what's your relationship to time? When are you when you're simply being? A man at the same homeless shelter answered these questions with, "Time? Who cares?"

In your journal, write down words that best describe your felt-sense of time when you're just being.

Isn't it interesting how, when you're experiencing being, thinking settles down, self-consciousness disappears, and with it your sense of time ceases? Time is irrelevant when you're just being—you're outside of past, present, and future, all of which are concepts that are dependent upon thinking. As you settle into just being, thinking and time slow down and may even stop. So, another description of yourself as being is that you are *an undeniable presence that's timeless and whole.*

Messenger #3: Lacking and Flawed Versus Perfect

When you're just being, is there anything that you need to make you any better or more perfect than you already are as being? How are you when you're simply being? Veterans, service members, people grieving or in pain, or people who are feeling just fine all respond similarly to this question. They all say that when they're absorbed in being, they don't feel that they are either lacking or flawed. They feel perfect just as they are as being.

In your journal, write down words that describe your felt-sense of need when you're just being.

When you're simply being, can you feel the perfection of being, just as it is? Can you feel how trying to acquire something can take you away from the feeling of being? So, another description of yourself as being is that you are *beyond need and feeling flawed or lacking, and perfect wholeness just as you are.*

Messenger #4: Confused and Disconnected Versus Connected

When you're just being, is there anything you need to know that would make you any more connected than you already are as being? What are you when you're simply being? One veteran replied, "I don't need to know anything to know *being.* I've known this feeling all my life. I'd just forgotten it in the midst of my pain."

In your journal, write down words that describe your felt-sense of needing to understand or feel connected when you're just being.

Whenever I open up a great book, whether it's the Bible, Koran, Bhagavad Gita, or *Jonathan Livingston Seagull,* the message is the same: "Just be, and know who and what you truly are." You don't need extra knowledge to recognize being. In fact, seeking knowledge can take you away from being. So, another description of yourself as being is that you are *an undeniable presence and complete wholeness, just as you are.*

Messenger #5: Incomplete Versus Complete

When you're just being, is there anything you need to do that by doing it would make you any more complete than you already are as being? Who are you when you're simply being? After hearing these questions, most people understand that they don't need to do anything special to be. They know that they can be at any time, anywhere. And they feel how being is a powerful source of well-being.

In your journal, write down words that describe your felt-sense of how you feel when you're just being.

Can you feel how being doesn't need any particular doing to be what and how it is? It's complete and whole just as it is. With all sincerity, a woman in a shelter said, "This practice with the five messengers has showed me my real home. Now I can deal with my homelessness." So, another description of yourself as being is that it's your true home. As being, *You're an undeniable presence that's complete and whole just as you are. You need to do nothing in order to be your complete wholeness.*

Being Human and Whole

A beautiful fact about being and wholeness is that they're basic elements of your being a human. When you're just being, you discover the wholeness that is your birthright. You discover that, as a human being, you're actually:

- *Spacious*, even as your need for maintaining and affirming healthy boundaries continues

- *Timeless*, even as your psychological need for time continues

- *Perfect*, even as your personal desires continue to arise

- *Connected*, even as your need to obtain objective knowledge and social connections continues

- *Complete*, even as your need for doing continues

Experiencing your basic being and wholeness doesn't depend on fixing or changing yourself. Your being is already and always spacious, timeless, perfect, connected, and complete. At your core, you're already and always healthy and whole. Experiencing your being throughout the day helps you stay connected to yourself and to your wholeness, which is what supports you in healing feelings of alienation, separation, and isolation.

PTSD disrupts your sense of wholeness. The symptoms can make you feel disconnected from yourself, your relationships, and the world. The practice of iRest helps you to remember your felt-sense of being and wholeness. The practice reconnects you to yourself and restores your ability to feel connected to others and the world. Through your practice of iRest, you learn to experience yourself as a unique and separate individual who is also interconnected with and not separate from all of life.

From the place inside yourself where you're always connected, whole, healthy, and harmonious, you can safely address your symptoms of PTSD. By first experiencing your inner being and wholeness, you put in place a foundation on which you can stand. Having a foundation to stand on allows you to address what does feel broken and is in need of fixing and changing.

Forgetting

I've shown you how your five special messengers can reveal your basic being and wholeness. Now allow me to show you how you forget your being and wholeness. The following practice demonstrates how your sense of being can get overpowered by the symptoms of PTSD, causing you to forget your wholeness. The practice also shows you how to maintain your sense of wholeness. This Forgetting and Remembering practice shows you that there's nothing wrong with *you*, even as you address symptoms of PTSD that reveal what is wrong and needs changing with your body and mind. Remember, the feeling that "something's wrong" doesn't mean something's wrong with you. Let me make sure this is crystal clear for you. The symptoms of PTSD that you're experiencing do need to be fixed and changed. But *you*—your basic being and wholeness—do not need to be fixed or changed. You are already and always whole and okay!

📓 🔊 Practice 3: Forgetting and Remembering

Lie or sit in a comfortable position. Open your senses to your surroundings... sound...color...light.... Open to the feeling of the environment around you... the touch of air on your skin...the sensations where your body touches the surface that's providing support...the feeling of your entire body...and your sense of simply being.... Take delight in not having to be anywhere...nothing to do...nowhere to go.... Simply enjoy the easy feeling of just being....

Welcome and enjoy the felt-sense of spacious timelessness that's present as you're just being...the felt-sense of feeling perfect...connected...complete...and whole as you're just being...the felt-sense of well-being, harmony, and peace that is present as you're just being....

Now, imagine that unexpectedly you experience a challenging life event. Someone angrily interacts with you. You fall and injure yourself. Or something goes wrong at home, work, or on the street.... In this moment the details of the event absorb your attention. You feel contracted and upset. You begin to feel that something's wrong and lose touch with your inner sense of being and wholeness.

Then, suppose that, before you're able to recover from this event, life knocks you down again. And, as you're getting up, it knocks you down again. Overwhelmed by the intensity of your experience, you completely lose touch with your inner sense of being and wholeness. Your ego gets the message that "something's wrong" and translates it to you as, *Something's wrong with me. There's something I need to do or know so I can feel whole again.*

Imagine that you try all sorts of things to feel better, but you continue to feel disconnected and confused. Then the thought comes, *Maybe there's something I need to know.* So you start reading books and seeking advice. When this fails, you continue to feel confused and disconnected. Then the thought comes, *Maybe there's something I need to acquire to recover my inner peace.* But this fails and you move even further away from your sense of wholeness. Then the thought appears: *If only I could have more time and more space I could figure this all out.* But when this fails, you now feel helpless, lacking, confused, and disconnected. You feel that you've run out of time in your capacity to heal yourself.

As you identify with these feelings, you experience yourself as broken, separate, isolated, confused, and powerless in your failures to experience the well-being that you once knew. You're exhausted from looking everywhere for healing and not finding it anywhere.

Then, one day, shattered and weary, you collapse into your chair. Having tried everything, you give up and momentarily fall into the experience of simply being. In this moment of being, your judging mind slows down. Your sense of wholeness breaks through, and you feel in yourself a sense of being that is spacious, timeless, perfect, connected, and whole just as it is, just as you really are in your essential wholeness of being.

You find yourself "home" again. Resting as being and reexperiencing your wholeness, you reconnect to your sense of peace and harmony. Now you remember. Resting here, you feel powerful again as your ego lets go of identifying with the thought, *Something's wrong with me*. As you remember your felt-sense of being, you feel a sense of your basic wholeness flowing through your body and mind. You take time to rest here—as being—feeling your underlying wholeness. With this feeling of wholeness, you know that you can now turn your attention to healing what's wrong from the place within yourself that's perfectly right. But before you turn to facing what's wrong and taking care of business, you take time to relax into being so that your body and mind can bathe in the refreshing waters of being that are your natural state of wholeness.

Before returning to your wide-awake state, take some time to fully relax into being.... Allow the sense of being to flow through your entire body and mind.... When you feel refreshed, open and close your eyes several times, welcoming in the world around you, while maintaining your felt-sense of being and wholeness as you move back into your daily life.

Being Home

The tools of iRest help you come back home to yourself. They teach you how to welcome "what is" in each moment. They help you address what needs changing and fixing in your body and mind. The practice of welcoming "what is" empowers you to reexperience your natural state of being and wholeness. Trying to fix and change what's wrong without first experiencing your being and wholeness is like rearranging the deck chairs on the *Titanic*. You might look and feel better on the surface, but you'll continue to suffer. Your ship is still going down! Welcoming and experiencing the five special messengers of being can help you awaken from your slumber of separation, pain, and confusion. These messengers are here to help you recover and experience your natural state of interconnected wholeness.

At first, you may think this approach is too simple. But a healing approach doesn't have to be complicated to work. Everyone I've worked with says the same thing when they recognize the healing power of being. One Vietnam veteran said, "It's so simple. Why didn't they give us this sooner? I wish I'd gotten this program when I first starting dealing with my PTSD."

Facing the symptoms of PTSD is not easy. Your symptoms, conditioning, and habitual ways of living can cloud your ability to recognize being. Being and wholeness are the doorways to true healing. The practices of iRest are designed to help you gain access to those doorways and overcome your conditioning, habits, and symptoms. These practices support you to remember being in the midst of your daily life, while eating, talking, playing, working, and even sleeping.

That's right, being and doing exist at the same time. But your symptoms of PTSD can make your experience of being and wholeness feel nonexistent. When you lose touch with being, you lose touch with other essential aspects of yourself, such as love, kindness, compassion, joy, and peace. The practices of iRest enable these aspects to blossom again, along with your underlying wholeness, as natural expressions of your being.

Moving Forward

In the coming chapters you'll learn how to experience your felt-sense of being and wholeness, as you also learn practices that address your symptoms of PTSD. The practices of iRest are designed to help you experience being and wholeness as always with you. Then, even in the midst of pain, loss, or suffering, you'll remain connected to your wholeness as you address what needs healing. Suffering does come to an end. Lasting peace and healing are yours for the asking.

Chapter 4

Affirming Your Resolutions

You are what your deep, driving intentions are. As your intentions are, so is your will. As your will is, so are your deeds. As your deeds are, so is your destiny.

—Upanishad text

Every healing journey starts with a resolution. Resolutions are vows you make to follow during your healing journey. Your inner vows set the path for your healing. Resolutions also nourish your motivation, patience, persistence, and perseverance—four qualities that enable you to stay on your healing journey. It's the strength of your resolutions that leads you to victory over PTSD. In the words of the Indian poet Kabir, "It is the intensity of your longing that does the work" (Bly 2004). With this in mind, the iRest Program for Healing PTSD begins with teaching you how to set your resolutions for healing. You'll learn to affirm your heartfelt mission, intention, and inner resource.

iRest Tool #1: Affirming Your Heartfelt Mission

Your *heartfelt* mission is the energy of life within you that gives rise to and sustains your inner felt sense of purpose, meaning, and value. It's the life force that's energizing every cell in your body and sustaining every breath you take, that gives you the energy to meet every challenge you face in life. Affirming your heartfelt mission puts you in touch with this dynamic force of life that can heal you through even your most challenging circumstances and symptoms of PTSD.

Your heartfelt mission is what motivates you to get out of bed each morning, no matter how you're feeling. I think of it as the mission that life has sent you on during your lifetime. As you live your life's mission, you feel in harmony with your place in the world. While I refer to it as *heartfelt mission*, others have named it their heartfelt path, heartfelt energy, heartfelt desire, or heartfelt purpose. Whatever you call it, it's the feeling within yourself that's moving you forward.

During this first stage of iRest, you acknowledge and welcome your heartfelt mission. Then you positively affirm it—not as a future possibility but as a statement of fact, true in this moment. So instead of saying, "May I trust life," or "I will trust life," you say: *I trust life in this and every moment.* Instead of saying, "May I feel my underlying health and wholeness in each moment," say: *I feel my underlying health and wholeness, in this and every moment.*

It's Always Now

It's important to state your resolutions in the present tense. Why? Because in reality, it's always *now*. Acknowledging this truth, the practice of iRest asks you to state your heartfelt mission as the truth of *this* moment. If you create your resolution by saying, "I hope to..." or "I will..." or "May I...," you put your resolutions on hold for some future date. You want support for your healing right now! So always state your resolution using *I am...* Even if you don't fully believe it in this moment, your act of saying your resolutions in the present tense makes them come alive as truth.

Your heartfelt mission is the core energy within you that provides motivation, purpose, and meaning in your life. The more you say your heartfelt mission, the more you feel yourself living *from* it. As you live from it, you feel how your heartfelt mission empowers you to be in harmony with yourself and with life. When you're in harmony with yourself and life, you experience yourself as a creative expression of life designed to live your life's purpose, in the same way every flower, tree, and blade of grass lives out its purpose in life's master plan. When you're deeply in touch with your heartfelt mission, you feel that you are living up to life's fullest potential.

Yes, I Can

Affirming your heartfelt mission every day allows it to be a strong healing force in your life. You'll know it's working when you catch yourself starting to fall into an old pattern of thinking, feeling, or acting. Instead of falling into your usual reaction, you'll take new actions based on your heartfelt mission. When you act from your heartfelt mission, you experience deepening trust and confidence in yourself. You'll come to know for certain that you can do whatever you say, including, *Yes, I can heal my PTSD*. Here's what Jim (a veteran with PTSD) said about finding his heartfelt mission:

> *I was helping a friend clean and organize her house. It was a windy and gray day, and I was feeling really miserable. When I was done helping her, I sat down in her backyard holding her puppy in my lap. John Lennon's song "Imagine" was playing on the radio as I began thinking about what my heartfelt mission might be. By and by, I began to feel really peaceful. I thought, So, this is what it's like to be with myself! It was really special. It was so serene and peaceful. I'd never been able to relax like that before. I can't explain how good it felt to just be with myself. After forty-four years, just to be with myself is amazing. I really like it. I now feel a sense of hope that I can trust life. Out of that experience came my heartfelt mission: I trust life and feel connected with myself.*

Working with Opposites

iRest teaches you to take time to welcome both the positive *and* negative feelings and thoughts that live in your body and mind. While positive feelings and thoughts support and advance your healing, negative feelings and thoughts can prevent or stall your healing. Therefore, it's important for you to learn to work with opposites of feeling and thought. In fact, it's just as important for you to learn how to work with the negative as it is for you to affirm the positive feelings and thoughts that come up as you heal. For instance, affirming, *I'm at peace and content with what each moment brings* helps you see more clearly when you're fighting with, and reacting to, what life *is* bringing to you. Affirming, *I'm deeply connected to myself, to others, and to life itself* helps you see more clearly the actions that make you feel disconnected from yourself, others, and life itself. Your ability to acknowledge both your positive and negative feelings and thoughts keeps your healing on track.

Your Negativity Bias

Like your early ancestors who lived millions of years ago, your DNA is biologically programmed with a *negativity bias*. This means your lower brain is hardwired to perceive the negative more readily than the positive in every situation. As a result, you perceive and respond to potential threats more readily than to potential positive situations (Graham 2013; Hanson 2009). According to your biological programming, it's better to mistake a stick for a snake, get frightened, and jump out of its way than to mistake a snake for a stick, step on it, and get bitten. While your biological programming causes you to more readily affirm the negative rather than the positive in any situation, iRest teaches you how to acknowledge the negative and turn it into a positive that can aid you in healing your PTSD. Negative thoughts and emotions—like shame and blame, self-judgment and self-rejection, fear and anxiety—are actually your friends. That's right. The practice of iRest teaches you how to welcome your negative emotions and thoughts as allies whose energy can be harnessed and turned into positive healing forces.

It's as important to think about and write down your positive heartfelt mission statements as it is to acknowledge and write down their negative opposites. You need to understand both the positive and the negative in order to heal your PTSD. With this in mind, make sure you also write down the negative opposites of your heartfelt mission statements in step 4 of the practice Affirming Your Heartfelt Mission, which follows. In chapters 7 and 8, you'll learn to engage these negatives as powerful friends that support you on your way to healing your PTSD.

📖 🔊 **Practice 4:** Affirming Your Heartfelt Mission

Here is an exercise to help you pinpoint your heartfelt mission.

1. In your journal, write down your answers to the following questions. Your answers will help you design your heartfelt mission.

   What are my core values? If I were fully living them—experiencing meaning, purpose, and value in my life—what would these core values be?

   What are the underlying themes of my life? If I were fully living them—feeling totally engaged in my life—what would these themes be?

2. After you write down the words that make up your core values and life themes, take time to sense how each word or phrase rings true in your body and mind. Then, arrange them in order of their importance to you.

3. Circle one, two, or three of the words that feel most important to you. Then, write them as a statement that represents your heartfelt mission. Finally, repeat this statement several times to embed it in your memory.

   Here are some examples of the heartfelt mission that others before you have discovered:

   - I am a vital, potent, and creative force.
   - I feel my underlying health and wholeness in every moment.
   - I trust life and am at peace with what each moment brings.
   - My will and the will of life are one and the same.
   - My thoughts, words, and actions agree and align with one another.
   - I am deeply connected to myself, to others, and to life.

4. As you consider your positive heartfelt mission, write down any negative opposites that arise in your mind. You'll learn, in detail, how to work with these negative opposites in chapters 7 and 8. For now, just note them in writing.

5. During your practice of iRest, as well as throughout your day, affirm your heartfelt mission by saying and feeling it as a statement of fact that you take to be true about yourself and your life.

iRest Tool #2: Affirming Your Intention

Intentions represent powerful internal statements that help you fulfill your heartfelt mission. Like a compass, intentions keep you on course so that you can accomplish your heartfelt mission. Like the banks of a river, your intentions keep you flowing in the right direction.

Intentions are made up of both short- and long-term vows that help you harness your desire to achieve specific outcomes or goals. You may set specific intentions to support you to stop smoking, to follow a special diet, or to live a particular lifestyle. Intentions can also focus on working with a specific emotion, belief, or issue that keeps coming up in your life. Intentions are what support you to complete your healing of PTSD. They keep your course straight and true, no matter your state of mind, no matter your inner or outer circumstances.

This Moment, with Feeling

Like your heartfelt mission, your intentions emerge from within you. These are statements you affirm with deep feeling and determination in the present moment. Instead of saying, "I will stop smoking," you affirm, *I'm a nonsmoker.* Instead of saying, "Can I practice iRest every day?" you affirm, *I practice iRest each and every day.* When you affirm your intentions, say what you mean and mean what you say. That way, they are your living reality, in this and every moment of your life.

Practice 5: Affirming Your Intention

Here is an exercise to help you pinpoint your intentions.

1. In your journal, write down your answers to the following questions. Your answers make up your intentions.

    What are the intentions that I wish to affirm today?

    What are the intentions that best support living my heartfelt mission today?

2. After you write down the words and phrases that make up your intentions, take time to sense how each word or phrase rings true in your body and mind. Then, arrange them in order of their importance to you.

3. Circle one, two, or three of the words or phrases that feel most important to you. Arrange them so that they form your intention. Then, repeat your intention several times to embed it in your memory.

Here are some examples of intentions:

- *I'm respectful of and maintain healthy boundaries with others and myself.*

- *I note when I'm reactive, and I respond appropriately.*

- *I'm kind and nonjudgmental toward others and myself.*

- *I practice iRest daily. iRest enriches every aspect of my life.*

- *My relationship with myself and others is a source of harmony and love.*

- *I show up on time.*

- *I speak my truth with kindness in each and every moment.*

4. As you consider your positive intentions, write down any negative opposites that may arise at the same time. You'll learn, in detail, how to work with these negative opposites in chapters 7 and 8. For now, just note them in writing.

5. It's helpful to find one or two words that best represent your intention. For instance, the intention, I say "yes" when I mean "yes," and I say "no" when I mean "no" can be summed up with one word: truth. The intention, I eat and drink for health, vitality, and energy can be summed up by the words energy and health. Find one or two words that best represent your intention.

6. During your practice of iRest, as well as throughout your day, and during your Day's Review (see Practice 40 in chapter 12), affirm your intentions as statements of fact that you take to be true about yourself, right now, in the present moment.

Affirm your intentions with deep feeling and certainty. Experience this deep feeling and certainty in your body *and* mind. Then, watch what happens when you're about to say yes when you really mean no, or when you're reaching for an unhealthy food. When harmful habits that don't serve your heartfelt mission come up, your intention will arise naturally as a self-correcting behavior that supports you in healing your PTSD and living your heartfelt mission.

> *Judy is homeless and suffering from PTSD from her military experiences. During her seventh iRest class she reported, "I have a lot of injuries and pain from my military service. A friend said that iRest might help me with my pain. I made my intention to listen to the iRest CD every night before going to sleep. I've been doing that for the last month. It's strange—I'm feeling great. Difficult situations that I used to fight and resist are now easier to let go of. I'm not fighting life like I used to. And the pain in my body is a lot less. My doctor says this class is really good for me. I agree. Through this practice, I've recovered a 'happy place' within myself that I thought I'd lost. I'm feeling connected with myself in a way I never could have imagined before doing iRest."*

iRest Tool #3: Affirming Your Inner Resource

You possess within yourself an *inner resource* that's designed to empower you to feel in control of and at ease with every experience you have during your life. Your inner resource is a place of refuge within you. It provides you with inner support on every step of your healing journey.

The practice of iRest helps you discover your inner resource as a feeling of constant well-being. iRest teaches you to tune in to your inner resource and weave it into every experience of your life, both positive *and* negative. You affirm your inner resource when you're feeling at peace and in harmony with life. You affirm your inner resource when you feel overwhelmed by an emotion, belief, or experience. You call on your inner resource when you feel the need to take a momentary time-out from what you're experiencing. Your inner resource empowers you to face every circumstance, accomplish your intentions, fulfill your heartfelt mission, and experience success in healing your PTSD.

During iRest, as in daily life, there are moments when you encounter negative messengers, such as fear and anxiety, or feelings of sadness, emptiness, or aloneness. At these times, it's helpful to have instant access to your inner resource. Your inner resource counters negative experiences with positive opposites. It enables you to remember that indestructible security, perfect wholeness, and resilient well-being are always available to you, no matter your situation.

> *Mary is a veteran with PTSD and has a history of sexual trauma. Returning to her fifth iRest class she reported, "I'm usually full of rage every day, all day long. Thinking about what my inner resource is, I've become aware of a place that I didn't even know was here inside me. I realize now I'd closed the door on it years ago. As I've been exploring my inner resource, I've begun to feel a happiness and joy I thought I'd lost forever. It's amazing to feel joy again after feeling so angry and hopeless. I've begun using my inner resource all the time.*
>
> *"Two days ago, my boss got really aggressive with me. In response, I did something that's totally out of character for me because I'm usually very combative. I asked him if he was angry with me. When he answered, 'Yes,' I just said, 'Oh, okay.' I even apologized to him for what I'd been doing that made him angry, which is something I never would have done before. I felt really good inside. I cherish this iRest practice. My inner resource is really helping me learn how to work with my anger."*

Similar to your heartfelt mission and intention, your inner resource helps you feel in control of your life. It enables you to deal with harmful emotions, thoughts, and situations. Your inner resource is a powerful friend that's always with you. Affirming and experiencing your inner resource over and over again, during every iRest practice, as well as throughout your day, reminds you that it's always with you, always supporting you. You want to be so in touch with your inner resource as a vital force that eventually you don't have to think about it. Ultimately, you want to experience your inner resource affirming itself, all day long, each and every moment of your life.

Frank is a veteran who, as a result of his PTSD, experiences road rage whenever a vehicle unexpectedly cuts in front of him. When asked about his inner resource he reported, "The other day, I was driving next to an 18-wheeler truck. All of the sudden, the driver of the truck cut in front of me, pulled into the left lane, and turned into a parking lot. Every ounce of my body wanted to follow and give him a piece of my mind. But my hands and body kept steering me toward home instead. I know I wouldn't have done that a year ago. In that moment, I realized I had a choice. That's when I knew my inner resource was working for me. I don't need to remember it. It's remembering me."

Your inner resource is already hardwired into your central nervous system. It's a positive force that enables you to counteract any negative experience you're falling prey to. All you have to do is recognize and affirm your inner resource in your conscious mind. The practice of iRest empowers you to recover and put back into place this natural resource you have inside yourself.

Carl is living in a homeless shelter, taking part in a weekly iRest class. During his fourth class he reported, "This shelter is crowded and noisy, so I've been going to my car and listening to the iRest CD that you gave us to use between our weekly classes. I've been feeling terrible pressure in my heart because of losing my job, being homeless, and now breaking up with my girlfriend. I've been listening to the iRest CD over and over, all week long. Every time I feel my inner resource, I calm down. Several nights ago, I looked up through my sunroof and saw the stars. I sat there for a long time, gazing at the stars and feeling my inner resource. Usually I'm high-strung. But I woke up the next day and my mind was totally clear. My body felt calm, and I found myself in the flow, just letting life be as it is. I continue to feel this way. I now know I can deal with my feelings in a way I never imagined before coming to this iRest class. My inner resource is going to help me for the rest of my life."

Take time to remember and affirm your inner resource during your practice of iRest and throughout your day. Then, like it was for Carl, your inner resource becomes your friend. Your inner resource is always present. It's a source of stability and strength that you can call on under any circumstance, negative or positive.

Practice 6: Experiencing Your Inner Resource

Here is an exercise to help you pinpoint your inner resource.

1. In your journal, write down your answers to the following question. Your answers make up your inner resource.

   When I feel a sense of well-being, peace, or ease of being, where and how do I feel this in my body?

2. After you write down the words and phrases that make up your inner resource, take time to sense how each word or phrase rings true in your body and mind. Then, arrange them in order of their importance to you.

3. Circle one, two, or three of the words or phrases that feel most important to you. Repeat these words and phrases several times to embed them into your memory as prompts that represent and activate your inner resource.

   Here are some words that others have used to represent their inner resource:

   - Secure
   - Connected
   - At ease
   - Comfortable
   - Content
   - Still
   - Clear
   - Grounded
   - Peaceful
   - Expansive
   - Open
   - Safe
   - Stable
   - Balanced
   - Resilient
   - Flowing
   - Well-being
   - Being

4. As you consider your inner resource, write down any negative opposites that may arise. You'll learn, in detail, how to work with these negative opposites in chapters 7 and 8. For now, just note them in your journal.

5. Then, during your practice of iRest, as well as throughout your day, consider and affirm your inner resource as an inner felt-sense that you take to be true. Allow your inner resource to be your trusted friend that accompanies you on every step of your journey through life.

Your inner resource is an internal felt-sense that you carry with you. It's unique to you. Like drawing water from a well, you draw strength and comfort from your inner resource. As you form your inner resource, reflect on people, animals, objects, and places that help you recall it. Also consider sounds, tastes, smells, and other qualities that help you access it. Your inner resource is a multidimensional experience that you can reach through many inner and outer pathways. Here are some feelings and images others have found helpful as they discovered their inner resource:

- Inner feelings of security, safety, strength, ease, and well-being
- A peaceful flowing stream
- A still pond by a gently falling waterfall
- A serene and beautiful meadow
- A room filled with my favorite things
- A special loved one or animal
- A person who has special meaning to me
- A symbol that has special meaning for me

Jim, a Gulf War veteran suffering from a traumatic brain injury and PTSD, experienced severe anxiety while undergoing a routine MRI. Unable to continue, he jumped out of the MRI machine and fled the hospital. As the doors closed behind him, he later reported to us, "I once again felt defeated by my PTSD." That same afternoon, Jim attended an iRest class at the military base, where he was being treated. During his iRest practice, Jim called to his inner resource as a support for working with his anxiety. That evening, Jim returned to the same hospital he'd been to earlier that day. During his next iRest class, he said that he sailed through the MRI by feeling his inner resource ring true throughout his entire body and mind. As he left the hospital that night, he reported, "I felt victorious. I was in control of my PTSD. It was no longer in control of me."

Like it was for Jim, your inner resource supports you in gaining control of your negative experiences. Gaining control of your negative experiences enables you to feel a sense of resiliency and self-mastery. That's vital to healing PTSD (Wilson, Friedman, and Lindy 2001). During iRest, you learn to welcome and navigate negative feelings as part of your natural healing process. You learn to take control of your experiences—from anxiety and fear to feeling out of control—by calling to your inner resource.

It's contrary, I know, but iRest teaches you how to feel comfortable and in control in situations when you feel out of control. It does this by building your capacity to welcome your experience as a flow of changing movements within your unchanging ground of awareness. This practice supports your ability to release destructive emotions and recognize healthy responses. Your ability to welcome everything just as it is, both the positive and negative, while experiencing your inner resource, builds your ability to successfully overcome PTSD (Wilson, Friedman, and Lindy 2001).

When you first discover your inner resource, it may feel like something you're making up in your imagination. It's important to feel your inner resource *in your body*, as a physical sensation. With practice, you'll be able to instantly feel your inner resource. Ultimately, the most powerful inner resource is the simple feeling of being, as discussed in chapter 3.

Practice 7: Inner Resource Meditation

Sit or lie down in a comfortable position. With your eyes gently open or closed, allow your senses to open to the sounds around you...the sensation of your body touching the surface that's supporting you...sensations in your jaw...ears...eyes...forehead and scalp...the back of your neck and shoulders.... Open to the relaxed heaviness of your arms...and hands...the gentle rise and release of your abdomen with each breath...the sensations in your hips...legs...feet...the sensation of your entire body...without thinking... just being with the sensations of your body....

Inner Resource

Now, bring your attention to your inner resource.... Allow your inner resource to emerge as a felt-sense within your body...sensing feelings that you associate with being secure and at ease...and a felt-sense of well-being.... Notice in your body where and how you feel sensations of well-being.... Notice the words you would use to describe what you're sensing.... Take your time.... Experience your inner resource of ease and well-being...and the words that describe what and how you're feeling.... Allow your entire body to experience your inner resource of ease and well-being.... Affirm to yourself that you can return to this place of well-being at any time during your day and life... whenever you feel the need to feel secure, calm, at ease...and the feeling of well-being.... Take your time being with the feeling of well-being for as long as you wish....

Integration

When it feels right, allow your eyes to open and close several times while also maintaining the felt-sense of your inner resource of ease and well-being....

And as you're ready to return to your eyes-open waking state of consciousness, allow your eyes to remain open while continuing to feel your inner resource.... Allow your body to stretch and move about as you continue to welcome feeling secure, at ease, and the sense of well-being.... Affirm to yourself that you can return to your inner resource at a moment's notice any time you experience the need to feel secure and at ease...any time you feel the need to experience your inner felt-sense of well-being....

The "Little Universe" Inside of You

While working as a journalist for *Newsweek*, Maziar Bahari was imprisoned in Iran and held in solitary confinement for three months. Maziar's father and sister had also been imprisoned and tortured by a previous Iranian regime. During his captivity, Maziar drew strength from recalling conversations he'd had with his father and sister about their time in prison, as well as by recalling times he spent with his fiancée and mother. These memories helped him create his own inner resource of well-being. His inner resource was infused with memories of love-inspired conversations and experiences he'd had in the past. By continuing to feel his inner resource, Maziar was able to keep his mind and body in control, regardless of the physical and emotional turmoil he experienced. This "little universe inside of me," as he called it, was the way he protected himself from the physical abuse he suffered while imprisoned. He was surprised by how powerful his little universe was, how it shielded him and kept him "feeling intact, whole, unbroken, and unharmed within" (Bahari 2011).

Every Day in Every Way

Like Maziar did, start your day, spend your day, and end each day by taking time to sense your heartfelt mission, intention, and inner resource. Pair these three resolutions of healing and support with different states that you experience throughout your day. Recall them when you're feeling relaxed. Recall them when you're experiencing stress. Experience them when you're happy, when you're sad, when you're angry, when you're peaceful, when you're depressed, and when you're feeling on top of the world. Recall them when you're lying down, sitting up, and walking around. Remember them when you're talking with another, in person or on the phone. Remember them when you're working, eating, or resting. Then, like good friends, they will be there when you most need them. And like good friends, they'll even come to you on their own, without you having to call them.

Moving Forward

For your heartfelt mission, intention, and inner resource to be fully empowered as tools for healing your PTSD, you need to affirm them as truths in your mind and feel them in your body. It is the same for the other seven tools of the iRest program. Every iRest tool depends on your ability to sense, feel, and experience them in both your mind and body. They also depend upon your ability to sense, feel, experience, and respond to the messengers in your body and mind.

Your ability to sense the presence of various messengers depends on your relationship with your body and mind. That's what the iRest practice will help you do. In the next chapter, you'll directly address, develop, and deepen your relationship with your mind and body with Practicing Bodysensing, iRest tool #4.

Chapter 5

Bodysensing

An anxious mind cannot exist in a relaxed body.

—Dr. Edmund Jacobson,
the developer of progressive
muscle relaxation

You perceive the world through your five senses. Your body registers every sight, sound, smell, taste, emotion, thought, or image as sensation. Sensation generates and shapes your inner environment, as well as your experience of the world around you. You perceive warm and cool, pleasure and pain, anger and calm, and more because your body translates these perceptions into physical sensation. You sense when you or another is happy or upset because you register sensations of joy or distress in your physical body. When you're happy, you feel light and at ease. When you experience a distressing situation, thought, image, or memory, your body translates these perceptions into physical signals that register throughout your body as sensations. When this occurs, you may feel your jaw clench and your heart, stomach, or gut contract.

Let me share a story with you about the perceptive powers of our bodies. In the early 1970s, I taught a weekly iRest class to a group of blind students. The students occupied separate apartments in a large building composed of a maze of corridors with fire doors located at each end. I was astonished at how rapidly these students could walk down any hallway, stop in front of a fire door, open it, and continue walking briskly down the next corridor. On several occasions while we were walking together on streets we'd not visited before, individual students described to me buildings that were several hundred feet to the right or left of us. The blind students were able to sense doors and buildings through highly developed sensory feedback that registered in their bodies as physical sensation. These students' ability to sense and respond to incoming sensory information enabled them to live with the world within and around them. These blind students had made friends with their bodies.

Your Body Is Your Friend

Your body naturally knows how to heal itself from trauma and PTSD. Indeed, it not only knows how to heal, it also wants to heal. PTSD symptoms are in fact your body's way of calling your attention to your PTSD. By tuning in and listening to your body, you can learn to heal and thrive, not just survive.

When trauma overloads your nervous system with too much incoming information, *dissociation* can occur. Dissociation is when you disengage from yourself. It's your body's natural way of defending against overwhelming information. During a traumatic event your mind draws away from, and numbs your body to, sensory information that's overloading your system. Your body then produces symptoms of PTSD, as messengers whose purpose is ultimately friendly: to remind you that there's information you were unable to process at the time of trauma that you need to return to. Dissociation and your PTSD symptoms are your body's way of helping you return to the information you were unable to process at the time of the trauma-inducing event.

That said, when you experience extended periods of post-traumatic stress, you can feel that your body is not your friend but an "enemy." Your body's assortment of symptoms, such as arousal, numbing, vigilance, avoidance, depression, anxiety, fear, anger, and insomnia, can feel like betrayals. The good news is that your symptoms of PTSD are your allies. They're here to guide you to, and along, your pathway of healing.

Your symptoms of PTSD are your body's way of telling you that you have undigested sensory information that you need to process. The practices of iRest are "good medicines" designed to help you fully digest this sensory information. Once digested, your body and mind can return to their natural state of health, wholeness, and well-being. The practices of iRest enhance your ability to sense, welcome, respond to, and heal the variety of sensory input that your body and mind need to digest. One of the finest practices to begin your process of healing is *bodysensing*.

iRest Tool #4: Practicing Bodysensing

The practice of bodysensing teaches you how to sense, locate, welcome, and respond to sensory information. Through regular use of bodysensing, you are able to achieve deep physical and mental relaxation, calm and soothe your central nervous system, and stimulate your body's natural healing forces.

With this iRest tool, you grow to appreciate your body as a rich source of valuable feedback and healing resources. Your body's feedback is calling for your attention in order to help you heal PTSD and restore your physical, psychological, and spiritual vitality.

Listen to Your Body's Voice

I once had a teacher who always began his class using a soft and soothing voice. As each class progressed, however, his voice grew louder and louder. By the end of each class, he was shouting at us. Curious to understand his teaching style, I inquired one day, "Why do you shout so loud?" His answer surprised me. "I'm a radio," he answered. "When I sense that you aren't listening, I turn up the volume. If I speak loudly enough, you'll surely understand what I'm saying."

Like this teacher, your body turns up its volume to get your attention whenever you haven't heard the subtle messages it's sending. Your PTSD symptoms are your body's way of shouting to get your attention. Therefore, it's helpful to learn to detect subtle cues so that you don't have to wait until your body has to shout for your attention. When you're able to respond to early stress symptoms, you won't have to experience the more distressing symptoms that would have come later.

The practice of iRest in general, and bodysensing specifically, awakens your capacity to locate and respond to the subtlest of messages your body is sending you. When you're able to respond to these subtle cues, you'll be able to take practical, positive actions long before your body shouts for your attention. As you recognize and understand the range of sensations that your body's constantly sending you, you gain access to important feedback. This feedback enables you to be a creative caretaker of your body and mind.

Your Body as Radiant Sensation

Your mind, working along with your eyes, imagines that your skin defines the boundary of your body. Your body is actually a field of sensation that extends beyond any border or boundary that your mind creates. In reality, your body has neither an absolute center nor a defined boundary. Your body is a field of radiant sensation that extends infinitely in all directions. The following exercise offers you the opportunity to experience this for yourself.

Practice 8: Sensing Your Hands

During the following practice, take time to pause to fully experience each segment of the exercise.

With your eyes open, begin examining your hands...palms...fingers... back of your hands.... Notice their shape...color...texture...lines...edges.... Notice hair...spots...scars...fingernails.... Notice the thoughts that come to your mind as you examine your hands....

Now close your eyes and feel your left hand.... Let go of thinking about your hand.... Experience the actual sensations that make up your left hand.... Feel sensations of pulsing...throbbing...radiating.... Notice your hand as a field of sensation.... Feel how far out this field of sensation reaches.... Don't go into thinking.... Keep feeling your left hand....

Now feel your right hand.... Experience the actual sensations that make up your right hand.... Feel sensations of pulsing...throbbing...radiating.... Notice your right hand as a field of sensation.... Feel how far out this field of sensation extends.... Don't go into thinking.... Keep feeling your right hand....

Now feel both hands simultaneously.... Take your time.... Don't go into thinking.... Allow the energy and aliveness of your hands to fully unfold in your awareness.... Feel your two hands as a field of sensation that extends out into the space....

65

Now open your eyes and keep feeling your hands.... Now close your eyes again while continuing to feel your hands.... Now begin to welcome sensations throughout the rest of your body. Feel your entire body as sensation.... Now open your eyes while you continue feeling your hands and body.... Look around you while continuing to feel your hands and body.... Before returning to your daily activities, take a few minutes and reflect on your experience. Then record your reflections in your journal.

Thinking Versus Feeling

Notice how, as you feel your hands, your thinking about them decreases. Then, notice how, as as you go into thinking about your hands, you go away from feeling your hands. In reality, you can't feel your body and think about it at the same time. You can do one, or the other, but not both at the same time.

This simple exercise is designed to reveal the powerful effect of feeling versus thinking. As you switch from thinking to feeling, thinking automatically slows down and you activate a natural relaxation response in your body. The longer you remain with body sensations, such as those of your hands, the more thinking slows down and the deeper the natural relaxation response will be throughout your body and mind. As another example, try the following exercise.

Practice 9: Peeling Away Tension

With your eyes open or closed, sense and feel your jaw.... Don't go into thinking...just sensing and feeling your jaw.... Notice how your jaw, mouth, and other parts of your body soften and relax as you continue sensing and feeling your jaw.... Notice how, as one layer of sensation is experienced, it dissolves and a next layer is revealed.... Keep attention in your jaw. As you do this, feel the progressive relaxation response that deepens over time. Notice how this relaxation response then migrates to other parts of your body.

Now sense your shoulders...without thinking...just sensing and feeling your shoulders.... Notice how your shoulders soften and relax as you stay with sensation without going into thinking.... Just as before, as one layer of sensation dissolves, the next layer of sensation is revealed.... Keep attention in your shoulders. As you do, feel the progressive relaxation response that deepens over time....

Feel free to continue engaging this practice with other parts of your body...your face...arms...torso...pelvis...legs...or with your entire body as a field of sensation.... Don't try to relax or dissolve tension.... Simply stay with sensation and experience how your body naturally lets go into an ever-deepening relaxation response....

When you're ready to return to your normal waking state of consciousness, allow your eyes to open and close several times as you begin stretching and moving your body...noticing the environment around you while continuing to feel your body....

Before returning to your daily activities, take a few minutes and reflect on your experience of the practice you just did. Then record your reflections in your journal.

Sense Your Body, Grow Your Brain

Every part of your body has a connection to your brain. Taking advantage of these connections, modern neurophysiologists use sophisticated equipment to stimulate nerves deep in your brain to produce relaxation in your body. By practicing iRest, you can also take advantage of these brain-body connections to achieve deep states of relaxation. During iRest, you generate deep relaxation by practicing bodysensing—systematically moving your attention throughout your body. This iRest tool stimulates these very same nerves that lie deep within your brain and produces profound changes in your physical body, brain structures, and emotional and mental states.

Bodysensing, and the other practices of iRest, work from the outside in (from your skin to your brain) to effect changes from the inside out (from your brain to your skin) so as to produce deep relaxation and physical release from tension, stress, and negative ways of thinking, feeling, and reacting. Research reveals that mindful meditation practices, such as iRest, produce structural changes in your brain that are involved with enhancing memory, learning, gaining perspective, and regulating your emotions and thoughts (Hölzel et al. 2009). By regularly practicing bodysensing, you create changes in the structure of your brain that soothe your nervous system. You can grow your capacity to respond rather than react to stimuli—and therefore heal your PTSD.

Relaxing into Your Greatness

iRest incorporates a number of approaches and techniques for inducing deep relaxation throughout your body and mind. These approaches and techniques include *progressive muscle relaxation, autogenics,* and the *relaxation response.*

Progressive Muscle Relaxation

Dr. Edmund Jacobson, who developed *progressive muscle relaxation* (PMR), discovered that tensing your muscles for a few seconds and then releasing them leads to the release of stress and muscle tension, an increase in relaxation throughout the entire body, and the recovery from a host of medical and psychological conditions (Jacobson 1938; Carlson and Hoyle 1993), including the following:

Decreases in:	Increases in:
Depression	Calmness
Fatigue	Clarity of thinking
Generalized anxiety	Concentration
Headaches	Creativity
High blood pressure	Emotional control
Insomnia	Energy
Irritable bowel	Feelings of joy and peace
Muscular tension	Inner balance
Negative emotions	Overall health
Pain	Restful sleep
Panic attacks	Self-esteem
Phobias	Spontaneity
Racing thoughts	
Stuttering	
Ulcerative colitis	

Practicing PMR helps you notice large and small differences between tension and relaxation in the muscles throughout your body. I was first introduced to PMR in 1970 during a twelve-week yoga class. The instructor used PMR during yoga nidra at the end of each class. I was amazed at the level of stress I was able to release and the depth of relaxation I was able to achieve in just a few minutes of practicing PMR. Now, when I teach PMR to students, I commonly hear how relaxed they feel and how deeply they sleep due to the amount of tension they shed as a result of practicing PMR during iRest.

Autogenics

Johannes Schultz and Wolfgang Luthe created *autogenics* (1969) as a method of producing profound relaxation and healing through mental suggestion. Autogenics training involves affirming mental directives, such as "Cool forehead," "Relaxed and heavy arms and legs," "Warm hands, belly, and feet," "Slow, calm, and regular heartbeat," and "Slow and rhythmic abdominal breathing." Research shows that affirming these and similar intentions during iRest bodysensing produces a profound relaxation response throughout your entire nervous system, increases your ability to discern internal feedback from your body and mind, and enables you to achieve a relaxed and receptive state in which healing spontaneously occurs (Stetter and Kupper 2002; Luthe and Schultz 1969).

The benefits of autogenics training are many and include:

Relaxation of your body and mind

Restful sleep

Relief from anxiety and fear

Reduced fatigue

Reduced tension in your muscles

Improved interpersonal relationships

Increased efficiency in your work

Relaxation Response

Bodysensing also takes advantage of Dr. Herbert Benson's pioneering research and technique called the *relaxation response* (2000). The technique involves assuming a comfortable position in a peaceful setting, while quieting the mind and mentally hearing and repeating to yourself an inner sound such as *ahhh* or *hmmm*. Any other sound that feels relaxing is also suitable.

Benson discovered that this approach brings about a deep calming reaction, resulting in:

Deeper breathing

Profound states of rest and relaxation

Decreased heart and breathing rate

Increased levels of brain waves that are associated with deep relaxation

Decrease in the stress hormone cortisol

Feelings of satisfaction, inner balance, and peace

Research shows that the long-term benefits of progressive relaxation, autogenics, the relaxation response, and other bodysensing approaches produce a *generalization effect*. That means the deep relaxation you experience through a regular practice of bodysensing can be extended to the rest of your daily life (Novey 2000). Here's the way the generalization effect impacts your life:

- The more you practice bodysensing, the more relaxed and at ease you feel in all your daily interactions with others and yourself.

- The more you practice, the more you decrease stress, anxiety, and fear.

- The more you practice, the more you increase your clarity of mind, your capacity for restful sleep, your ability to thoughtfully respond rather than mindlessly react, and your ease of being throughout your daily life.

Your Friend for Life

As with each stage of iRest, the motto guiding your practice of bodysensing is *Every day, a little and often.* I invite you to practice bodysensing daily in small, frequent doses. Make it your regular habit to scan your body and release unnecessary tension. Do quick scans while working at your desk or computer, talking on the phone, driving to the grocery store, engaging in conversation, or while being with yourself. Weave bodysensing into all your daily activities, throughout each and every day of your life. Bodysensing is a tool that's always ready to help you relax into your wholeness and well-being, no matter your circumstance. By using this powerful tool you can feel, as I do, that bodysensing is your friend for life.

What follow are some guidelines and exercises that will support your practice of bodysensing. These bodysensing exercises combine the techniques of progressive muscle relaxation, autogenics, and the relaxation response. Experiment to find the practice that suits you best in the moment. Let your body tell you when it's time to try a different one. Feel free to mix and match exercises so that you make them your own. Welcome to bodysensing!

Guidelines for Practicing Bodysensing

- At first, practice bodysensing at least *20 minutes per day.* Over time, as you gain skill, you'll find that it takes just a few minutes to experience deep relaxation. Having a consistent daily practice of bodysensing develops your ability to quickly attain deep relaxation throughout your body and mind.

- Practice regularly, so that eventually you can perform bodysensing free of a script.

- For your practice, it's best to find a quiet place where you won't be disturbed.

- Assume a comfortable position on a sofa, bed, reclining chair, or on the floor. Your entire body, including your head and neck, should be supported. When lying down, place a pillow beneath your knees to help relax your lower back. Sitting is preferable to lying down when you're feeling tired or sleepy.

- Loosen your belt or any tight clothing. If possible, take off your shoes, watch, glasses, contact lenses, and jewelry.

- Always begin by affirming your heartfelt mission, intention, and inner resource. Put aside the concerns of the day. Assume a "let go and let it happen" attitude.

- As you experience sensations of relaxation, affirm to yourself, *I'm relaxed and at ease. I can let go now.* Feel free to find a phrase that feels right to you.

- Throughout bodysensing, maintain your focus on sensation. If your attention wanders, bring it back to the sensation of the particular muscle group you're working with.

Guidelines for Practicing Progressive Muscle Relaxation

Progressive muscle relaxation involves tensing and relaxing different muscle groups of your body.

- Tighten each muscle group without straining for 5 to 10 seconds while concentrating on the buildup of tension and sensation.

- Then, fully release all tension and give yourself 10 to 20 seconds to completely relax. Be aware of and enjoy the sensation of relaxation and letting go in contrast to how it feels when you're tensing the muscles.

- Allow all other muscles in your body to remain relaxed while you're tensing and releasing a particular muscle group.

- Tense and relax each muscle group once. But if a particular area feels especially tight, you can tense-release it two or three times, waiting 10 to 20 seconds between each cycle.

Practice 10: Progressive Muscle Relaxation

Begin your practice of PMR by adjusting your body so that you feel completely supported by the surface on which you're resting…. With your eyes open or closed, allow your senses to open to the sounds around you…the feeling of the air on your skin…scanning your body and releasing any unnecessary tension…welcoming sounds…sensations…and relaxing into being at ease throughout your entire body and mind….

Heartfelt Mission

Take a few moments and reflect on your heartfelt mission…. This is your mission that gives your life purpose, meaning, and value…. Perhaps your mission is your desire for peace, ease, or inner harmony…. Take a few moments now to experience and be with your deepest heartfelt mission….

Intention

Bring to mind your intention for this practice of bodysensing…or for what helps you affirm and live your heartfelt mission…. Your intention might be to relax…to rest…to be at ease…. Whatever your intention is, fully welcome and affirm it with your entire body and mind….

Inner Resource

Bring your attention to your inner resource…to sensations of being at peace… to feeling secure and grounded…to feeling at ease…. Experience your inner resource as a felt-sense of well-being that you can turn to whenever you need to take time out to feel secure and at ease….

Breathing

Now inhale deeply…. Then, while exhaling slowly through your nose, imagine tension throughout your body flowing away…. Repeat this breath pattern and tension release three times….

PMR

Now, stretch, tighten, and release the following muscle groups in your body….

Stretch open your jaw and mouth as wide as you can.... Hold your jaw and mouth open as wide as you can for the next 5 to 10 seconds while you welcome sensation throughout the muscles of your jaw...lips...tongue...and mouth.... Then, release your jaw and allow your mouth to close so that your lips are lightly touching.... Gently move your jaw back and forth.... Now completely let go and relax.... Allow your upper and lower jaw to slightly separate...jaw muscles soft and at ease....

Close your eyes and tense all the muscles of your lips...cheeks...nose... and eyes. Hold.... Now, while exhaling, relax completely.... Keep sensing your lips...cheeks...nose...eyes...all your facial muscles and skin...soft and at ease....

Tense the muscles of your forehead and ears by raising your eyebrows and furrowing your brow.... Hold.... Now, while exhaling, relax completely... sensing your forehead muscles soft and at ease...your inner and outer ears open to sensation and sound....

Tense the muscles throughout your neck.... Focus only on tensing the muscles of your neck while everything else in your body remains relaxed and at ease.... Hold.... Now, while exhaling, relax completely while sensing your neck muscles soft and at ease....

Tense your shoulders by raising them up toward your ears. Hold.... Now, while exhaling, completely release, relax, and sense your shoulders....

Tighten the muscles of your shoulder blades by bringing them together behind your back.... Keep everything else in your body completely relaxed and at ease.... Hold.... Now, while exhaling, relax completely.... Just experience sensation...without going into thinking....

Tighten your biceps by drawing your forearms toward your shoulders, making a muscle with both arms.... Hold.... Now, while exhaling, relax completely....

Tighten your triceps by extending your arms out straight while locking your elbows.... Hold.... Now, while exhaling, relax completely....

Clench your fists.... Hold for 5 to 10 seconds.... Now, while exhaling, release and rest at ease...no thinking...just welcoming sensation....

Tighten the muscles of your chest...ribs...and upper back.... Hold.... Now, while exhaling, relax completely, allowing unnecessary tension throughout your chest and back to release and dissolve away....

Tighten your belly...side...and back muscles.... Hold.... Now, while exhaling, relax completely.... Feel warm waves of sensation spreading throughout your abdomen and lower back....

Tighten the muscles throughout your pelvis and buttocks.... Hold.... Now, while exhaling, relax completely....

Squeeze and tense the muscles in your hips...thighs...hamstrings...and knees...no thinking...everything else completely at ease.... Hold.... Now, while exhaling, relax completely....

Tighten your calf and shin muscles.... Hold.... Now, while exhaling, relax completely....

Tighten your ankles, feet, and toes.... Hold.... Now, while exhaling, relax completely....

Progressively tighten your entire body...toes...feet...ankles...forelegs...knees...thighs...hips...buttocks...pelvis...belly...chest...lower back... upper back...fingers...hands...arms...shoulders...shoulder blades...neck... scalp...forehead...eyes...nose...cheeks...mouth...jaw.... Hold your entire body in tension for 10 to 20 seconds.... Now, while exhaling, release your entire body.... Welcome waves of sensation and deep relaxation spreading throughout your entire body...no thinking...just sensation...the body as a field of radiant sensation....

Scan your body for residues of tension.... If particular areas remain tight or tense, repeat one or two tense-release cycles at your leisure for these groups of muscles....

Continue sensing waves of warmth...sensation...deep relaxation... spreading throughout your body...jaw...ears...cheeks...nose...eyes...forehead...scalp...neck...arms...hands and fingers...chest...abdomen...upper and lower back...pelvis...hips...thighs...forelegs...ankles...feet and toes.... Feel warm sensation flowing throughout your body...every muscle releasing and relaxing...from your mouth to your toes...deep inside...and out to the skin...the entire body a field of radiant sensation....

Lie here as long as it feels right.... Welcome sensations of well-being... peace...and the ease of simply being.... Enjoy the pleasure of sensation... ease...and deep relaxation flowing throughout your body....

Completion

Rest here as long as it feels right.... When you're ready, in your own rhythm and timing, gently open and close your eyes several times.... Sense your surroundings while also welcoming deep relaxation...ease...and well-being throughout your body.... Welcome in your inner resource and heartfelt mission along with feelings of ease and well-being throughout your body....

Affirm to yourself that as you go about your life...walking...talking...eating... working...playing...and even sleeping...sensations of deep relaxation and well-being are accompanying you in every moment....

At your leisure, and when you're ready, come fully back to your eyes-open state of wakefulness.... Be grateful for taking this time for yourself, for health...for your healing...and for your practice of iRest....

Before returning to your daily activities, or moving on to the next practice, take a few minutes and reflect on the PMR practice you just did. Then record your reflections in your journal.

⬛ ◖ Practice 11: Bodysensing with Autogenics

Begin your practice of bodysensing with autogenics by adjusting your body so that you feel completely supported by the surface on which you're resting.... Open your senses...scanning your body and releasing any unnecessary tension.... Welcome sounds...sensations...and the feeling of being at ease throughout your entire body and mind....

Heartfelt Mission

Take a few moments and reflect on your heartfelt mission...the felt-sense of life living you that gives your life purpose, meaning, and value....

Intention

Bring to mind your intention for this practice of bodysensing and for what helps you affirm and live your heartfelt mission.... Your intention might be to stay present throughout this practice or to welcome a particular messenger in your body or mind.... Whatever your intention, fully welcome and affirm it with your entire body and mind....

Inner Resource

Bring your attention to your inner resource...to sensations of being at ease... secure...grounded.... Experience your inner resource as a felt-sense of well-being that you can turn to whenever you need to take time to feel secure and at ease....

Bodysensing with Autogenics

Now, begin sensing your body with the understanding that whatever you experience is perfect just as it is.... Be aware of sensations in your jaw... mouth...tongue.... Give up thinking and welcome sensation in the jaw and mouth, just as they are....

Sense your left ear...right ear...welcoming both ears simultaneously as radiant sensation....

Sense your cheeks...nose...nostrils...the flow of sensation inside both nostrils....

Sense your left eye...right eye...the feeling of both eyes simultaneously as radiant sensation.... Give up analyzing.... Simply feel your way....

Sense your forehead...cool and at ease...scalp...back of the head... neck...inside the throat...at rest and at ease....

Sense your left shoulder and shoulder blade...left upper arm...elbow... forearm...wrist...hand and fingers...the entire left arm...heavy...relaxed...at ease....

Sense your right shoulder and shoulder blade...right upper arm... elbow...forearm...wrist...hand and fingers...the entire right arm...heavy... relaxed...at ease....

Give up thinking, and welcome both arms and hands simultaneously as radiant sensation....

Bring attention into the upper chest...middle chest...abdomen...upper back...middle back...lower back...the entire torso...front and back...as radiant sensation.... Let go of thinking.... Just feel your way...your entire torso heavy and relaxed...warm and at ease....

Sense your pelvis...left buttock and hip...left thigh...knee...foreleg... calf...ankle...foot...toes...the entire left leg...heavy...relaxed...at ease... aware and attentive...relaxed and at ease....

Sense your right buttock and hip...thigh...knee...foreleg...calf...ankle... foot...toes...the entire right leg...heavy...relaxed...at ease....

Welcome both hips...legs...and feet simultaneously as radiant sensation...both legs heavy...relaxed...and at ease....

Sense the entire front of the body...back of the body...left side of the body...right side of the body...sensation inside the body...sensation on the surface of the body...the entire body relaxed...and at ease...as radiant sensation....

Feel yourself as an observer, as the spacious openness of awareness, in which all of these sensations are coming and going.... Sense your breathing and heartbeat...slow...steady...regular...your entire body and mind relaxed and at ease....

Well-Being

Feel sensations of well-being...peace...relaxation...spreading throughout your entire body...with every exhalation, sensations of warmth...ease...and well-being radiating throughout your body...face...torso...arms and hands... legs and feet.... Sense well-being...peace...and deep relaxation throughout your entire body...the body a field of radiant sensation....

Allow your ears to open to the sounds of your body breathing...to the natural sounds that your body is making during exhalation and inhalation.... Give your undivided attention to feeling your body as a field of sensation, while hearing the natural sounds of your body breathing. As you listen, welcome in the felt-sense of your inner resource and feelings of security, ease, and your body letting go into deep relaxation and well-being....

Completion

Rest here as long as it feels right for you.... When you're ready, gently open and close your eyes several times.... Reorient yourself to your surroundings while sensing deep relaxation, ease, and well-being throughout your body.... Sense your inner resource and heartfelt mission along with feelings of ease and well-being throughout your body.... Affirm to yourself that as you go about your life walking, talking, eating, working, playing, and even sleeping...sensations of deep relaxation and well-being are accompanying you in every moment....

At your leisure, when you're ready, come fully back to your eyes-open state of waking consciousness...grateful for taking this time for yourself, for your health...for your healing...and for your practice of bodysensing.... Before returning to your daily activities, take a few minutes and reflect on the practice you just did. Then record your reflections in your journal.

Moving Forward

As you develop your practice of bodysensing, it's normal to perceive your body as radiant sensation and currents of energy flowing throughout and expanding beyond the borders of your physical body. As you do, it's common to also become aware of the expansion and release of your abdomen and chest, and your body breathing through its cycles of inhalation and exhalation. It's natural, then, to turn your attention to the iRest tool of *breathsensing*, the subject of the next chapter.

Chapter 6

Breathing for Life

Grow steady in your breath and you will quickly discover peace of mind.

—Yogavasishtha, 10th century CE

Each day, you take an average of 24,000 breaths. And through those breaths, you take in more than 10,000 gallons of air. On days when you're highly active, you can take in twenty-five times this amount of air! The amount and the way you breathe plays a central role in every physical activity you engage. Your breath is closely linked to your digestive processes, cellular growth, muscle tone, blood flow, and heartbeat. Your breath is also closely linked to your thoughts, feelings, and mental and emotional states. Whether you're depressed, excited, angry, or calm, your breathing patterns change to match your mental and emotional state. When your breathing patterns are disorganized, your emotions and thoughts will become unsteady. Similarly, when your breathing patterns are rhythmic, your emotions and thoughts will be steadier. When your thoughts and emotions are stable, you can settle more easily into experiencing your inner resources of ease, security, and well-being (Fried 1987, 1990; Fried et al. 1983; Grossman 1983; Rama and Hymes 1979).

iRest Tool #5: Practicing Breathsensing

Understanding the role your breath plays in your daily life, as well as the way you breathe, can directly assist you in healing your PTSD. In this chapter, I'll be sharing with you the iRest practice called *breathsensing*. Breathsensing teaches you to pay attention to how you're breathing. Your ability to pay attention to your breathing does the following:

- Enhances your ability to sense, welcome, and respond to internal and external information

- Helps you to take the actions that keep you feeling in harmony with yourself and life

- Increases your physical and mental relaxation

- Soothes and strengthens your central nervous system

- Stimulates your body's natural healing forces

Your Healing Breath

Your breath is one of the most powerful healing resources that you have readily available to you. Therefore, to heal your PTSD, it's important that you learn to work in partnership with your breath. A classic symptom of PTSD is a pattern of short, shallow, and irregular upper-chest breathing. Upper-chest breathing is your body's way of increasing oxygen, boosting energy, and activating your *fight-flight-freeze response*. This provides the energy necessary for you to respond to stressful and traumatic events. However, long-term shallow chest breathing—which occurs with continued trauma, stress, and PTSD—produces patterns of chronic hyperventilation, decreased *respiratory sinus arrhythmia* (RSA), and lowered *heart-rate variability* (HRV), which I'll define for you in the next section.

Shallow chest breathing, hyperventilation, and decreased RSA and HRV are designed to stimulate your kidneys to release *cortisol*. Cortisol is a hormone that increases your blood sugar for quick energy. It also activates your fight-flight-freeze response, so that you can quickly respond to life-threatening situations. That's the good news. The bad news is that cortisol, when overproduced as a result of chronic stress or PTSD, increases your body's vulnerability to disease; makes you feel tired, fearful, and depressed; and causes you to become overly reactive to your inner and outer environments.

On the other hand, deep, slow, and rhythmic whole-body breathing patterns involve all of your body's breathing muscles, not just those in the chest. Whole-body breathing patterns activate your *rest-renew-heal response* and help you to feel relaxed and in control of your experience. Taking long exhalations while breathing with your whole body:

- Reduces anxiety and fear

- Increases your relaxation response

- Supports your immune system

- Releases healing hormones into your system

In this case, instead of cortisol, your body produces *serotonin* and *oxytocin*, your feel-good hormones. These hormones reduce pain, support feelings of well-being and loving-kindness, and assist you in feeling connected with yourself and the world (Zak 2012; Kosfeld et al. 2005; Miller 1991).

Respiratory Sinus Arrhythmia and Heart Rate Variability

Now, let me explain *respiratory sinus arrhythmia* and *heart rate variability*. As you exhale, your heart slows down, your rest-renew-heal response is stimulated, oxytocin and serotonin are released, and your entire body goes into relaxation. As you inhale, your heart speeds up, your fight-flight-freeze response is activated, cortisol is released, and your entire body is energized. To promote health, nature has designed your exhalation to be slightly longer than your inhalation. On average, healthy adults and children have an exhalation that is one and a half times longer than their inhalation. For example, while reading a book, eating, or talking, if your inhalation is two seconds long, your exhalation is probably around three seconds long. This interaction of breathing and heart rate is called respiratory sinus arrhythmia (RSA) and heart rate variability (HRV). Healthy RSA and HRV support physical and mental health, and help your body and mind to be resilient, so that you can survive times of stress and thrive in your daily life (Miller 1991).

Symptoms of PTSD include shallow, upper-chest breathing whereby your inhalations become equal to, or longer than, your exhalations. Studies show that upper-chest breathing with longer inhalations than exhalations decreases RSA and HRV and increases anxiety, fear, panic, and depression. Decreased RSA and HRV also result in increases of blood pressure and the risk of heart attack, stroke, and heart disease. On the other hand, slow, deep, whole-body breathing, whereby your exhalations are longer than your inhalations, increases RSA and HRV. Increased RSA and HRV lead to reductions in the psychological and physical symptoms listed in table 1 (Angelone and Coulter 1964; Hirsch and Bishop 1981; Ross and Steptoe 1980; Eckberg, Kifle, and Roberts 1980; Clarke 1981; Eckholdt et al. 1976; Stanescu et al. 1981; Trzebski, Raczkowska, and Kubin 1978; Yongue, Porges, and McCabe 1980; Hincle, Carver, and Plakun 1972; Johnston 1980).

Table 1. The Effects of Whole-Body Versus Upper-Chest Breathing

Whole-Body Breathing Slow, rhythmic breathing	Upper-Chest Breathing Shallow, irregular breathing
Enhanced respiratory sinus arrhythmia (RSA) Enhanced heart rate variability (HRV)	Reduced respiratory sinus arrhythmia (RSA) Reduced heart rate variability (HRV)
Indicator of good health	Indicator of health risk
Psychological Effects	
Increases emotional stability and resiliency	Decreases emotional stability and resiliency
Increases calmness, relaxation, and confidence	Increases excitation and shyness
Increases physical and intellectual activity	Decreases physical and intellectual activity
Increases sense of control	Decreases sense of control
Decreases perceived stress	Increases perceived stress
Decreases anxiety and fear	Increases anxiety and fear

Physical Effects	
Increases rest-renew-heal response	Increases fight-flight-freeze response
Decreases cortisol and increases oxytocin and serotonin	Increases cortisol
Decreases heart-lung stress and risk of heart attack or stroke	Increases heart-lung stress and risk of heart attack or stroke
Decreases blood sugar levels	Increases blood sugar levels
Decreases muscle tension	Increases muscle tension
Decreases fatigue, need for sleep, and physical pain	Increases fatigue, need for sleep, and physical pain
Increases blood and oxygen to brain, heart, and tissues	Decreases blood and oxygen to brain, heart, and tissues
Increases relaxation response	Increases stress response
Decreases blood pressure	Increases blood pressure
Decreases type-A behavior (characterized by aggressiveness, restlessness, and a strong sense of time urgency; associated with coronary heart disease)	Increases type-A behavior

Mindful Breathing

The iRest practice of breathsensing offers you a host of benefits for leading a healthy life. Breathsensing nourishes your ability to concentrate. It supports your central nervous system in maintaining a healthy balance between your fight-flight-freeze and rest-renew-heal responses. Breathsensing helps you release tension and feel at ease in your mind and body. It also improves your ability to sense and respond to the messengers that are constantly delivering information to you from your body and mind. Your improved ability to sense and respond to this information supports you to be responsive, compassionate, and caring toward yourself and others (Graham 2013; Hanson 2009).

During the practice of iRest, you're guided to note and follow your breath. Noting and following your breath develops your ability to focus on the experience of your body's natural cycles of inhalation and exhalation. While noting and following your breath, you're asked to not change your breathing patterns in any way. You simply note, follow, and experience your breath as a natural flow of sensation. By paying attention to your breathing in this way, you increase your ability to experience and understand the flows of breath, sensation, and energy in your physical body.

Mindful breathing—paying attention to your breathing patterns—helps you focus your attention on, and be in tune with, your breath as a moment-to-moment flow of sensation, energy, and feedback. There are many ways of breathing mindfully. You can be aware of the touch of air at the entrance of your nostrils. You can note your belly expanding and contracting with each inhalation and exhalation. You can experience the relaxation response that comes with every exhalation. Or you can note the movement of breath as a flow of sensation and energy in different parts of your body.

For instance, as you inhale and your belly expands, you can experience sensation expanding upward and outward in your body. As you exhale and your belly releases, you can experience sensation flowing downward and inward in your body. As you attend to these and other sensations in your body as you breathe, you'll discover flows of sensation that are moving in every direction: downward, upward, forward, backward, sideways, and diagonally. Paying attention to your breathing focuses your attention, releases thinking, relaxes your mind and body, and supports your ability to gain perspective over your thoughts and emotions. Having the ability to gain perspective enables you to sense and respond to subtle messengers of sensation, which helps you feel in control and in harmony with yourself and the world.

Experiencing Breathsensing

Breathsensing is a vital tool in your tool belt of iRest practices for healing PTSD. In the following pages of this chapter, I offer you three different breathsensing practices. Try each one so that you can develop a range of experiences with them. Once you have participated in these exercises, you'll have a clearer understanding of which practice is best for the particular PTSD symptom you're experiencing. As time passes, you'll come to know which practice is best for you at any given moment.

First, try breathsensing during specific iRest practice periods. Then, integrate it into your daily routines. Like bodysensing, breathsensing is something you can practice all day long, each and every day of your life, for the rest of your life.

One important guideline to keep in mind as you practice breathsensing is to fully enter into the experience of your breath. Rather than thinking about your breath, note, feel, follow, and experience it. Feel yourself completely engaged by the sensation of each breath. You'll be amazed by how just a few minutes of breathsensing can leave you feeling grounded and refreshed—and able to respond to the moment, no matter your circumstance.

Practice 12: Noticing Flows of Inhalation and Exhalation

In this practice, you note and follow the natural flows of inhalation and exhalation within your body. You don't interfere with your breathing pattern in any way. As you simply note and follow your breath, notice the natural sense of well-being that's present. In a place where you won't be disturbed, take 5 to 10 minutes to experience this practice.

Sit or lie down in a comfortable position. Adjust your body so that you feel completely supported by the surface on which you're resting.... With your eyes gently open or closed, allow your senses to open.... Welcome sounds... sensations...the touch of air on your skin...the sensations of your body where it touches the surface it's resting on.... Notice the feeling of letting go into being at ease throughout your entire body and mind....

Bring attention to sensations in your jaw...mouth...eyes...forehead... neck...shoulders...arms...palms...chest...belly...upper and lower back... pelvis...hips...legs...feet.... Welcome your entire body as a field of radiant sensation...front and back...left and right sides...inside and out.... Welcome your entire body as a radiant field of sensation....

Noticing Your Body Breathing

Bring attention to the sensation of your body breathing...just noting...just feeling...without going into thinking.... Notice your body breathing...the sensation and feeling of each inhalation and exhalation as it comes and goes....

Noticing the Expanding and Releasing of Your Belly, Midsection, and Chest

As your body inhales, note your belly, midsection, and chest expanding, while feeling yourself settling, relaxing, and letting go....

As your body exhales, note your chest, midsection, and belly releasing... while feeling yourself settling, relaxing, and letting go....

If your mind wanders, gently and nonjudgmentally bring it back to noting the gentle expanding and releasing of your whole body with each inhalation and exhalation....

Notice sensations as your body breathes in...and out...sensations of expanding and releasing with each breath....

Welcome and nourish the feeling of your inner resource of well-being as you continue to note your breath coming in, and going out...every cell in your body welcoming the feeling of well-being with each breath....

Continue noting, welcoming, and experiencing your body breathing... the sensation of your body expanding...and releasing...with each breath.... Notice your entire body and mind relaxing with each breath...feeling at ease...peaceful...grounded.... Allow each breath to invite in your inner resource of well-being, peace, and ease.... Remain here as long as you feel comfortable, noting and being at ease with each breath....

Completion

When you're ready, allow your eyes to slowly open and close several times.... Sense the surface that's supporting your body...the feeling of the environment around you...sounds...objects...the sensations of your body...sensations of well-being...emotions...thoughts that are present....

As you're ready, with your eyes open, feel yourself present to this moment...aware of your body breathing...your inner resource...and sensations of well-being, peace, and ease as you come fully back to your wide-awake state of mind and body...present to this moment.

Practice 12: Follow-Up

Take a few minutes and reflect on what you've just experienced. How does your body feel now, as opposed to how it felt at the start of this practice? How does your mind feel? What's happening with your thinking mind? Do you feel calmer, more relaxed, and more at ease than you did when you began this practice? Did you experience particular thoughts, feelings, or emotions as you practiced noticing your breathing? Can you imagine how you might use this practice "on the fly," in the midst of your daily life? If so, make it your intention to practice breathsensing when it occurs to you or when you feel the need to relax, rest, and restore yourself. If helpful, record your reflections in your journal.

Practice 13: Noticing Flows of Sensation and Energy

All the movement in your body—thoughts, emotions, sensations, images, et cetera—are actually flows of energy. Your breathing patterns are also flows of energy. At first, these flows may be subtle and challenging to feel. With practice, however, these flows become easy to feel and experience.

In this practice, you're invited to note and experience your breathing as flows of sensation and energy. In a place where you won't be disturbed, set aside 5 to 10 minutes to experience this practice.

Sit or lie down in a comfortable position. With your eyes gently open or closed, allow your senses to open to the sounds around you...the touch of air on your skin...the sensations where your body touches the surface that it's resting on.... Notice the feeling of letting go into being at rest and at ease throughout your entire body and mind....

Bring attention to sensations in your jaw...mouth...eyes...forehead... neck...shoulders...arms...palms...chest...belly...upper and lower back... pelvis...hips...legs...feet.... Welcome your entire body as a field of radiant sensation...front and back...left and right sides...inside and out.... Welcome your entire body as a radiant field of sensation....

Noting Flows of Sensation and Energy

Bring your attention to your body breathing...inhaling...belly, midsection, and chest rising.... Feel your entire body expanding...and letting go into the surface that's supporting you...expanding and letting go...relaxed... grounded...at ease....

Bring attention to your body breathing...exhaling...belly, midsection, and chest releasing...your body letting go into the surface that's supporting you...releasing...relaxing...grounded...and at ease....

With each exhalation, sense a gentle flow of sensation and energy moving up the back of your body...flowing along the back of your legs... back of your spine...back of your neck...and up and out through the top of your head.... With each exhalation sense a flow of sensation and energy up the back of your body as your body settles ever more deeply into the surface that's supporting you....

With each inhalation, sense a gentle flow of sensation and energy traveling down the front of your body...flowing down through the top of your head...throat...chest...belly...pelvis...legs and feet.... With each inhalation sense a flow of sensation and energy traveling down the front of your body as your body settles ever more deeply into the surface that's supporting you....

Notice this circulating current of sensation and energy...with each inhalation, sensation and energy flowing down the front of your body from head to toes...with each exhalation, sensation and energy flowing up the back of your body from heels to head....

Welcome and nourish the feeling of your inner resource of well-being as you continue noting your body breathing...every cell in your body welcoming the feeling of well-being with each breath....

Continue noting and experiencing this circular flow of sensation and energy with each breath...your body settling...relaxing...grounded...at ease...inviting in your inner resource of well-being, peace, and ease with every breath...remaining here as long as you feel comfortable....

Completion

When you're ready, allow your eyes to slowly open and close several times.... Sense the surface that's supporting your body...the feeling of the environment around you...sounds...objects...the sensations of your body...emotions...thoughts...and the feeling of well-being....

As you're ready, with your eyes open, feel yourself present to this moment...aware of your body breathing...your inner resource...and sensations of well-being, peace, and ease as you come fully back to your wide-awake state of mind and body...present to this moment.

Practice 13: Follow-Up

Take a few minutes and reflect on what you've just experienced. What particular thoughts, feelings, or emotions came to your attention as you practiced the breathing? Were you able to sense them, and your breath, as flows of energy? Are you able to welcome them as messengers that are here to help you find harmony in your life? Can you imagine how you might practice the noticing of flows of energy and sensation "on the fly," in the midst of your daily life? If so, make it your intention to work with this breathsensing practice whenever it occurs to you, or when you feel the need to relax, rest, and restore yourself. If helpful, record your reflections in your journal.

Practice 14: Breath Counting

As well as noting and following the flows of sensation and energy of your breath, the iRest practice of breathsensing also invites you to spend time counting your breaths. This practice is particularly useful in training your mind to concentrate and pay attention. Attention and concentration training develops and strengthens your ability to stay with a task for the time needed to accomplish a particular goal. To succeed at anything, be it healing your PTSD, getting a good night's sleep, finishing a work-related task, deepening your relationship with yourself or someone you care about, or developing a sense of well-being, your mind needs to possess the ability to remain focused for as long as it's necessary to accomplish your goal. *Breath counting* helps strengthen your ability to remain undistracted for as long as a task needs your complete attention.

When counting your breaths, you'll find yourself becoming distracted by random thoughts. Each time this occurs, gently and nonjudgmentally refocus and begin counting from the beginning again. Distraction and refocusing are natural and occur over and over again during breath counting, as they do in daily life. Each time you refocus, you're strengthening your mind's ability to remain undistracted for longer periods of time both in breath counting and in your daily life. With time and patience, you'll find yourself able to remain present and undistracted even as distracting thoughts arise.

At first, breath counting, like other breathsensing practices, can feel challenging. It's like trying to rub your stomach and pat your head at the same time. But I encourage you to stay the course with the practice. In time, with patience and practice, you'll discover the physical, mental, and spiritual benefits that come as a result of doing this simple practice. Staying focused and attentive, as well as patient and persistent, are key to healing your PTSD.

Sit or lie down in a comfortable position. With your eyes open or closed, allow your senses to open to the sounds around you...the touch of air on your skin...the sensations where your body touches the surface that it's resting on.... Notice the feeling of letting go into being at ease throughout your entire body and mind....

Bring attention to sensations in your jaw...mouth...eyes...forehead... neck...shoulders...arms...palms...chest...belly...upper and lower back... pelvis...hips...legs...feet.... Welcome your entire body as a field of radiant sensation...front and back...left and right sides...inside and out.... Welcome your entire body as a field of radiant sensation....

Bring attention to your body breathing...without changing your breathing in any way.... Notice your body breathing and the natural flows of sensation...in your nostrils...throat...chest...midsection...belly.... Notice your belly gently rising and expanding as air flows in, and then gently releasing as air flows out....

Breath Counting

Continue sensing your belly expanding and releasing with each breath while counting your breaths from 1 to 11.... Count like this: *Inhaling, belly expanding 1; exhaling, belly releasing 1...inhaling, belly expanding 2; exhaling, belly releasing 2...and so on....* Notice your body breathing, the sensation of the breath, and the movement of the belly while counting from 1 to 11...present, awake, and aware of each count....

When you recognize that you've been distracted by a thought, gently and nonjudgmentally bring your attention back to your body breathing...starting over again with your counting at 1 each time you find that you've become distracted...your mind present and attentive to counting each breath as your belly expands...and releases....

Continue counting while sensing and releasing tension that's present in your mouth...ears...eyes...scalp...shoulders...arms and palms...torso...legs and feet.... Be naturally drawn to areas of sensation throughout your body... sensing the breath...the expansion and release of the belly...at ease... awake...and present to the count of each breath and the gentle rise and release of your belly....

Welcome and nourish the sensation of your inner resource of well-being, peace, and ease as you continue counting...every cell in your body welcoming the feeling of well-being with each breath...with each count....

Now let counting gently stop.... Stay with the flows of sensation and energy that are present as your body breathes...not thinking...not trying to figure anything out...simply experiencing flows of sensation and energy....

Completion

When you're ready, allow your eyes to slowly open and close several times.... Sense the surface that's supporting your body...the feeling of the environment around you...sounds...objects...the sensations of your body...emotions...thoughts...and the feeling of well-being....

As you're ready, with your eyes open, feel yourself present to this moment...aware of your body breathing...your inner resource...and sensations of well-being, peace, and ease as you come fully back to your wide-awake state of mind and body...present to this moment....

Practice 14: Follow-Up

Take a few minutes and reflect on what you've just experienced. Can you feel how the movement of attention is like a muscle that you can strengthen through a practice like breath counting? Did any particular thoughts, judgments, or emotions come to your attention as you practiced? Can you welcome the thoughts, judgments, and emotions as messengers that are here to help you find harmony in your life? Can you imagine how you might use this practice "on the fly," in the midst of your daily life? If so, make it your intention to practice breath counting when it occurs to you, or when you feel the need to relax, rest, and restore yourself. If helpful, record your reflections in your journal.

Sensing the Pulse of Life Within Yourself

Every molecule in your body is pulsating with energy. While PTSD can disconnect you from feeling this natural pulse of life, bodysensing and breathsensing are practices designed to reconnect you to this amazing vibration of life. They enable you to experience the flows of sensation and energy within your body.

During bodysensing and breathsensing, you take time to feel and nourish the pulse of life. Your intention, heartfelt mission, and inner resource represent this pulse of life that gives purpose, motivation, and meaning to your life. Practice breathsensing and bodysensing, and affirm your intention, heartfelt mission, and inner resource regularly during your day to experience the flows of breath, sensation, and energy—along with feelings of peace, ease, and well-being—throughout every moment of your life. As you do these practices, you're building the foundation that will enable you to heal your PTSD and thrive in your life.

Moving Forward

As you become aware of the flows of sensation and energy within yourself through bodysensing and breathsensing, it's natural to encounter feelings and emotions that are present in your body. Sensing feeling and emotion is a signal that you've entered into the territory that's addressed by iRest tool #6, Welcoming Opposites of Feeling and Emotion, in the next chapter.

Chapter 7

Welcoming Opposites of Feeling and Emotion

As I learned to stay with the truth of what I was feeling, I felt liberated each time I experienced my emotion without looking away.

—Lucy, iRest participant

PTSD and its accompanying sets of symptoms activate brain functions that can ramp up your feelings and emotions, and make you feel out of control in your life and relationships. In this chapter, you'll learn the role your feelings and emotions play in healing your PTSD.

Defining Feelings and Emotions

First, let me define *feelings* and *emotions*.

Feelings, such as cool/warm, dull/sharp, rough/smooth, and so on, are the physical sensations that make up your emotions. Feelings describe your emotions. Feelings are like ingredients cooking in a pot.

Emotions, such as courageous/fearful, calm/anxious, peaceful/angry, joyful/grieving, and so on, are the physical states that arise in response to circumstances and relationships. Emotions describe these physical states. Emotions are like the pot that holds the ingredients.

You need both the pot and the ingredients to make a stew, just as you need both feelings and emotions in order to fully welcome and describe a particular experience you're having. For instance, you're having a particular experience when you say, "I'm anxious." Anxious is how you're describing the group of sensations you're having, such as sweaty palms, dry throat, contractions in your gut, and worrisome thoughts. You may say, "I'm angry," which describes a group of sensations you're experiencing, such as a tight throat, flushed cheeks, racing heartbeat, and shallow breathing.

In order to heal your PTSD, you have to be able to welcome the feelings you're experiencing as well as name the emotions that best describe your experience.

iRest Tool #6: Welcoming Opposites of Feeling and Emotion

The intensity of the feelings and emotions that accompany your PTSD can hold you hostage when their stormy waters flow through your body and mind. This is because they activate your nervous system, which releases chemicals into your bloodstream that can take your body minutes, hours, and even days to fully process. iRest tool #6, Welcoming Opposites of Feeling and Emotion, is designed to help you sail through these stormy seas. This tool enhances your ability to respond to your feelings and emotions with actions that leave you feeling empowered and capable of handling any situation that arises in your life.

Be Fearless

Unresolved feelings and emotions can cause you to experience great physical and mental suffering and disharmony. When suffering and disharmony arise, what you may most want to do is label your feelings and emotions as the *enemy*. You may want to refuse your feelings and emotions when they come uninvited into your awareness. But refusing, as a way to cope with your feelings and emotions, doesn't work. It only postpones facing what you need to face. Every feeling and emotion you deny will always return, because every feeling and emotion is a messenger trying to deliver important information to you. When correctly understood, this information helps you respond to your circumstances and relationships in ways that foster health, healing, and well-being.

I invite you to pause here a moment to fully consider the fact that your feelings and emotions are necessary to healing your PTSD and living a full life. They're not your enemies. They're your friends! Your feelings and emotions want to be welcomed. Your feelings and emotions want to be seen, heard, and felt. If you don't learn how to welcome and attend to them, you'll continue to feel stuck, unable to heal your PTSD, and incapable of moving forward in your life.

The iRest practice of Welcoming Opposites of Feeling and Emotion is designed to show you how to stay connected with and respond to your feelings and emotions. That's right, *stay connected with* and *respond to* your feelings and emotions even when you'd rather run from them. This requires courage on your part. The more you stay with and respond to your feelings and emotions, the more fearless you'll feel when experiencing them. This practice teaches you how to be fearless when you're afraid. It teaches you how to feel secure when you're insecure, and relaxed when you're anxious. It teaches you how to be calm when you're angry, hopeful when you're depressed, and strong when you're feeling vulnerable or exposed.

Alan was in command of a vehicle that entered Baghdad as part of the first wave of troops, whose mission it was to liberate the city. As his vehicle drove into the city, it was met by crowds of citizens who, shouting and singing, poured out of buildings from every direction. As men and women surrounded and began to climb onto his vehicle, Alan didn't experience the joy of these citizens. Instead, he experienced the adrenaline rushing through his body, designed to keep him focused and alert to danger. Even as his superiors issued orders to hold fire, all Alan could feel was fear for his life and the desire to protect the men under his command.

Upon returning stateside, all Alan could recall from this mission was the fear he'd felt during those hours and months he'd spent in Iraq on heightened alert. As he practiced iRest, he learned to welcome his fear as a messenger. He also learned to welcome the opposite of fear—which, in this circumstance, is joy. As a result, he was able, for the first time, to experience the joy and celebration that had been present the day he'd entered Baghdad. He was also able to welcome every feeling of joy and celebration he'd denied himself since returning from his tour of duty.

Before practicing iRest, joy and celebration only reminded Alan of his feelings of fear and hypervigilance. After practicing iRest, he was able to experience joy separate from fear. This was a major step for Alan in healing his PTSD and moving forward in his life.

Your Emotions Are Messengers

At their core, feelings and emotions are feedback mechanisms. I call these feedback mechanisms *messengers*. These messengers are designed by nature to provide you with the information necessary to help you survive *and* thrive. For example, when you mistakenly touch a hot stove, pain arrives as a messenger to let you know you're in danger of burning your hand. Frustration arrives as a messenger when you've missed your plane and you need to consider a new plan of action that fits the new situation.

Your emotions and feelings are messengers that provide you with information regarding the ever-changing nature of reality within and around you. In and of themselves, feelings and emotions are neither good nor bad. They're neither right nor wrong. They simply provide information. Avoiding or reacting to your feelings and emotions blocks your ability to accurately respond to the world around and within you.

From the point of view of iRest, every feeling and emotion is designed by nature to help you get what you need. The iRest tool Welcoming Opposites of Feeling and Emotion teaches you how to welcome every feeling and emotion that comes your way as a messenger. Then, it shows you how to use the information that these messengers deliver to successfully navigate your way through every situation you encounter, so that you can get what you need, heal your PTSD, and thrive in your life.

Opening to a World of Infinite Possibilities

PTSD is your "friend." I understand that relating to PTSD as your ally may be hard to do when you're being tossed around by the rough waves of the feelings and emotions that are the symptoms of your PTSD. However, it's true. Your symptoms do not arise to cause you harm. Instead, they arise to get your attention, so that you can process them and heal your PTSD. iRest tool #6 invites you to turn inward in order to process and heal the feelings and emotions related to your PTSD. When you don't turn inward, you'll feel stuck and adrift by the waves of feelings and emotions associated with your PTSD.

Your experience of being stuck and adrift is your brain's way of getting your attention. That's right, your brain's designed to hold you captive. It does this so that you can attend to feelings and emotions that need your attention. Your brain does this through a variety of functions that make up your *focusing network*. Your focusing network gets your attention through various functions that include your senses, brain, and mental thinking processes. (Graham 2013; Carlson 2012).

Through the practice of Welcoming Opposites of Feeling and Emotion, you learn to shift your attention from one feeling or emotion to its opposite. This process of welcoming opposites shifts you from being stuck in your focusing network and moves you into the *defocusing network* of your brain. Your defocusing network enables you to recognize actions that empower you in your life and reconnect you with your felt-sense of wholeness (chapter 3) and the world of *infinite possibilities*. In the world of infinite possibilities, you can gain insight and healing that was otherwise unavailable to you when you were stuck. By shifting between opposites, while also experiencing your wholeness, you unlearn old patterns of reactive behavior and rewire new coping strategies into your brain that help you heal your PTSD (Graham 2013; Gerdes 2008; Segal 2007).

Practice 15: Experiencing Your Focusing and Defocusing Networks

In order to feel what it's like to shift between your focusing and defocusing networks, try the following practice. As you're listening, be sure to pause when you feel the need to take more time. This will allow you to fully experience each segment of the practice. Have your journal handy.

With your eyes open, welcome the environment and sounds around you...the touch of air on your skin...the sensations where your body touches the surface that's supporting it....

Bring your attention to an object that's out in front of you. Direct your attention to this object alone. Exclude all other objects that are around you and focus only on this one object.

Focus on the object's size...color...shape...and form.... Note particular thoughts you have about it....

Now, take in all the objects around you without focusing on any particular object, color, shape, or form.... Allow your attention to relax and defocus.... Soften your eyes.... Instead of looking with your eyes, sense from your heart as you take in all of the objects around you.... Sense and feel the space all around you...out in front...to your right and left...behind you.... Sense all these directions at once.... Feel like you're looking everywhere, without focusing on anything specific....

Now shift your attention back to the particular object you were first focusing on.... Bring it into sharp focus....

Then soften your eyes and feel yourself looking everywhere again.... Defocus your attention.... Don't focus on anything specific....

Go back and forth several times, focusing and defocusing your attention, and experience the effect this has on your body and mind....

Now try the same exercise with your eyes closed.... Sense an internal object...a sensation, an emotion, or a thought.... Focus your attention on this internal object alone.... Then shift your attention so that you feel like you're looking everywhere, without focusing on anything specific.... Then shift your attention back to a particular internal object...then feel yourself looking everywhere again.... Go back and forth several times, focusing and defocusing your attention with your eyes closed, and experience the effect this has on your body and mind....

Completion

When you're ready, allow your eyes to slowly open and close several times while feeling yourself present to this moment...aware of your inner resource... and sensations of well-being, peace, and ease...as you come fully back to your wide-awake state of mind and body....

When you're ready, take a few moments to write down words that describe what you experience when you shift your attention between being focused and defocused.

The iRest practice above teaches you how to actively engage your focusing and defocusing networks. This practice also teaches you how to weave your focusing and defocusing networks with Welcoming Opposites of Feeling and Emotion. Practicing in this way is a powerful exercise for transforming and healing PTSD. It will also give you the ability to heal and transform the way you think about and respond to the world within and around you.

Peace Is Yours for the Asking

Every feeling and emotion moves through a natural cycle of birth, growth, stability, decay, and dissolution. The degree to which you're able to welcome, experience, and allow your feelings and emotions to go through this natural life cycle is directly related to the degree to which you're able to feel fully engaged in your life and relationships. When you deny your feelings and emotions, peace and well-being remain out of your reach. When you welcome and allow your full range of feelings and emotions, you're able to recognize and experience lasting peace and well-being. Fearlessness and peace spread throughout your life when you're no longer afraid of experiencing fear *or* joy. When you're open to experiencing all of your feelings and emotions, anxiety and fear no longer control your life. Self-judgment loses its grip. Self-love, kindness, and compassion blossom. Here's what one participant reported when she was finally able to welcome her feelings and emotions during iRest:

> When I started practicing iRest, little did I know that the practice would ask me to face all of my emotions about the things I'd seen and done—things I never wanted to feel or think about. Through the iRest practice, I discovered that I had to face and feel them. I had to invite in my fear, anxiety, shame, guilt, and embarrassment. Each time I felt one of my emotions, my heart would pound. I felt vulnerable and afraid. I'd tried to avoid my emotions. But

that hadn't worked. I wondered, "How many of my emotions will I have to feel before I'm done? Is this ever going to end?"

So, what good came of this practice? As I learned to stay with the truth of what I was feeling, I felt liberated each time I experienced my emotion without looking away. As a result, I'm more at ease and comfortable with myself.

During iRest, parts of myself that I'd rejected, that had made me feel separate—my anger, shame, guilt, and embarrassment—came knocking on my door saying, "Let me in! Stop rejecting me. I am you!" So I let these parts in, and now I understand what it means to welcome messengers that are trying to deliver a message. During iRest, things that I'd rejected, including myself, came knocking on my door, inviting me to let them in. Letting them in has allowed me to finally feel whole again. Now I know what to do when a negative feeling shows up: I welcome it and do what it asks. I'm not perfect at welcoming and responding yet, but I'm learning.

Engaging Your Feelings and Emotions

Take time to experience the following five practices, which have to do with engaging your feelings and emotions. Each is designed to hone your ability to welcome and respond to every feeling or emotion that arises within or around you.

Practice 16: Welcoming Your Feelings and Emotions

When you encounter a feeling or emotion, your first task is to welcome and experience the feeling and emotion as a body sensation. Then, note where you experience this sensation in your physical body and how it's affecting your breathing. Have your journal handy.

With your eyes open or closed, welcome the environment and sounds around you...the touch of air on your skin...the sensations where your body touches the surface that's supporting it....

Experience the feeling and mood of your body.... Locate a feeling or emotion that's present.... Stay with what you're experiencing without going into memory or thinking.... Sense where and how you experience this feeling or emotion in your body....

Now ask: *Where do I feel this feeling or emotion in my body?... Is it in my belly, chest, throat, head, arms, or legs?...*

How would I describe this feeling or emotion that I'm experiencing?... What is its shape, form, color?... Is it solid or vaporous?... Does it appear as an object, animal, plant, or person?... Is it small or large?... As I experience it, do I feel tense or relaxed?... Heavy or light?...

Stay with your experience just as it is, whatever it is, and however it appears to you...while noticing where and how you're breathing. Are you breathing in your belly, midsection, or chest?... Is your breathing long, deep, and slow...or short, shallow, and quick?...

Now ask yourself: *Do I have any judgments about this particular feeling or emotion?... If so, what are they and how and where do I feel them in my body?...*

Describe your feelings and emotions to yourself in as many ways as you can.... Then come back to simply experiencing the felt-sense of this feeling or emotion...taking a few moments to simply experience the sensations that are present in your body that *are* this feeling or emotion...

When you're ready, allow your eyes to slowly open and close several times.... Sense the surface that's supporting your body...the feeling of the environment around you...sounds...objects...the sensations of your body... feelings...emotions...thoughts...and the feeling of well-being....

With your eyes open, feel yourself present to this moment, while sensing your inner resource...sensations of well-being, peace, and ease...present to this moment and your wide-awake state of mind and body....

When you're ready, write down your descriptions in your journal. Describing what you feel is part of the process of welcoming. It helps you gain perspective and break free of being entangled in the feeling and emotion that's present.

It's important to take time to welcome, experience, and describe the feelings and emotions arising within you. This keeps you in the present moment and forms the foundation that prepares you for the practices that follow.

Now that you've located and are experiencing the presence of feelings and emotions in your body, try the following practice.

Practice 17: Proactively Engaging Feelings and Emotions

With your eyes open or closed, welcome the environment and sounds around you...the touch of air on your skin...the sensations where your body touches the surface that's supporting it....

Take a few moments to experience the feeling and mood of your body.... As you're doing this, locate a feeling or emotion that's present...sensing where and how you experience this feeling or emotion in your body.... Now, imagine this feeling or emotion walking in through a door, or stepping into a meadow.... Go with the first image that appears in your imagination....

What does your feeling or emotion look like?... What is its shape, form, color, size?... Is it formless, or does it take the shape of a mineral, rock, plant, animal, or person?... If it's a human being, how old is it, and how is it dressed?... Take a few moments and simply welcome, with your imagination, the shape and form your feeling or emotion takes....

Now imagine this feeling or emotion standing or sitting in a chair at a comfortable distance in front of you.... You're going to ask your feeling or emotion three questions.... First, you'll ask it your question. Then, you'll imagine yourself as the feeling or emotion speaking the answer back to you. The three questions you'll ask in a moment are:

What do you want?

What do you need?

What action are you asking me to take?

Now, face your feeling or emotion and ask it, *What do you want?*... Now, imagine you are your feeling or emotion speaking the answer. Listen to what it has to say....

Next, ask it, *What do you need?*... Now, imagine you are your feeling or emotion speaking the answer. Listen to what it has to say....

Next, ask it, *What action are you asking me to take?*... Now, imagine you are your feeling or emotion speaking the answer. Listen to what it has to say....

Take a few moments to reflect on what you're now experiencing in your body and mind....

When you're ready, take time to write down in your journal your reflections and the answers you discovered from doing this practice. Any actions you've discovered that you need to take become intentions. When you set an intention, be sure to follow through with it in your daily life. Following through with your actions and intentions builds self-trust and self-esteem, important ingredients in your journey of healing your PTSD.

Remember, every feeling and emotion is a messenger delivering information and asking you to take an action. Actions can include speaking with someone, writing a letter, taking time to be with yourself, or simply taking time with your feelings and emotions. Here's an example of what can happen when you take time to welcome your feelings and emotions:

David was angry and sad. As a consequence of his PTSD, many of David's relationships had fallen away during the past several years, including his relationship with his son. During an iRest session, he took time to sense his body for feelings and emotions that were present. His attention was immediately drawn to a feeling in his throat that he described as dense, thick, and contracted. He reported that he'd tried all sorts of ways "to heal it, but it keeps coming back, and I don't know what it wants."

I asked him to close his eyes and imagine the sensations in his throat walking in through a door. Then, I asked him to describe what the sensation in his throat looked like. Without hesitation he answered, "A bear." I asked him to ask the bear the three questions about want, need, and actions, and to respond as if he were the bear answering each question. Taking his time he responded, "I want you to stop and listen to me. I need you to pay attention to me or I'm going to keep growling and bothering you until you do. You need to call your son and make amends." David opened his eyes with new understanding about what he'd been avoiding the past two years.

Amazingly, David, right then and there in my office, took out his cell phone, called his son, and proceeded to have the beginning of what would be a complete reconciliation with his son. By listening to his feelings and emotions, David took an action that enabled him to feel empowered and in control of his life.

Using your active imagination is a powerful way of working with your feelings and emotions. Imagining them allows you the opportunity to speak with them as if you're interacting with an actual person.

It's most important to discover the actions you need to take in response to each feeling and emotion that you experience. Then, by taking action, your feelings and emotions will have delivered their messages and can go on their way. Keep in mind during each and every step toward healing your PTSD that *every* feeling and emotion you experience is a messenger, inviting you to take an action. Taking these actions empowers you!

Welcoming Opposites

Every feeling and emotion comes paired with its opposite. Hot can't exist without cold. Fear can't exist without courage. Sadness can't exist without happiness, and conflict can't exist without its opposite, peace. PTSD and its symptoms stay around when you're unable to fully experience opposites of feeling and emotion.

When you resist fully experiencing your anxiety, fear, grief, or help-lessness, you deny the experience of their opposites: peace, courage, joy, and confidence. When you experience only one half of a pair of oppo-sites—grief, for instance, but not joy; anger, but not calm; or shame, but not confidence—you remain stuck in your one-sided encounter. You become unstuck when you open to experiencing opposites of both feeling and emotion.

During the practice of iRest, you're invited to welcome the opposites of feelings and emotions in connection with your PTSD. You can, for instance, welcome your feelings of pain or discomfort, and then invite their opposites—pleasure and comfort—into your body. You then swing back and forth between these feelings. After doing this for a few minutes, you then experience both feelings at the same time. You approach wel-coming opposites of emotions in this same way. For example, you may experience the emotion of anger or helplessness, and then explore the opposite of calm or confidence. Or you may experience the emotions of sadness, despair, or fear—and then explore their opposites of happiness, joy, and courage.

When you work with welcoming opposites, you explore where you experience feelings and emotions in particular areas of your body. For instance, the legs and pelvis are often associated with feelings of fear and safety, insecurity and security, and ungroundedness and groundedness. The belly is often associated with power and powerlessness, and helplessness and confidence, while the heart is linked to kindness and judgment. As you move back and forth between pairs of opposites, you also note the sensations that arise in their associated bodily areas. Welcoming opposites of feeling and emotion enables you to be connected to yourself. Welcoming opposites also allows you to take the actions that the feeling or emotion is asking you to take in order to feel empowered in your life. These actions you're prompted to take are called *right actions* because they come from the truth of your inner self. Taking right action helps you connect to your intention, heartfelt mission, and inner resource; helps you heal your PTSD; and helps you experience your underlying wholeness and well-being.

iRest teaches you how to welcome opposites of your experiences so that you can directly experience the core part of yourself—wholeness—that's never injured by traumatic events, that always remains whole and healthy. The iRest program helps you shift from identifying with what feels broken and in need of healing within you to what always remains whole and healthy. This frees you to relate differently to your past. It heals your physical, mental, and emotional pain, along with feelings of loss, grief, and helplessness. By working with opposites of feeling and emotion, you reclaim your ability to feel seen, heard, and connected. And you recover the sense of belonging, meaning, purpose, and value in your life.

Identifying Opposites of Feeling and Emotion

In order to personalize your practice of iRest, take out your journal and write down opposites of feeling and emotion that you associate with your PTSD. Note specific ones that you're struggling with in your life, or those you wish to work with for whatever reason. Once written down, you can draw on these paired opposites of feeling and emotion as you enter your practice of iRest.

Writing Down Opposites of Feeling

Here are some examples to help you pinpoint feelings that are meaningful to you. Don't limit yourself to just this list when considering your choices. Feel free to find your own words that best describe your feelings—in this way, you tailor your practice to your own life experience.

Alert	Floating	Sensitive
At ease	Grounded	Sharp
Awake	Hard	Sinking
Bright	Heavy	Sleepy
Broad	Hot	Smooth
Clear	Lethargic	Soft
Closed	Light	Spacious
Cold	Loose	Superficial
Comfort	Narrow	Tense
Confused	Numb	Thick
Constricted	Open	Thin
Cool	Painful	Tight
Deep	Pleasant	Ungrounded
Dim	Pleasurable	Unpleasant
Discomfort	Prickly	Warm
Dull	Relaxed	

Choose several feelings and their opposites that describe the sensations that you are or have been experiencing. Use the list here or come up with your own words. Record them in your journal.

Writing Down Opposites of Emotion

Here are examples to help you pinpoint emotions that are meaningful to you. There's no need to limit yourself to just this list when considering your choices. Find your own words to best describe your emotions—in this way, you tailor your practice to your own needs.

Abandoned	Frightened	Mellow
Aggressive	Frustrated	Numb
Agitated	Generous	Passive
Anxious	Grateful	Peaceful
Ashamed	Guilty	Perplexed
Assured	Happy	Potent
Boisterous	Harsh	Powerful
Bored	Hateful	Proud
Calm	Helpful	Resentful
Caring	Helpless	Responsive
Composed	Impotent	Rigid
Confident	Included	Sad
Delighted	Innocent	Safe
Depressed	Insecure	Satisfied
Disgusted	Interested	Secure
Enraged	Joyful	Sensitive
Exhausted	Kind	Shy
Fearless	Listless	Sneering
Flexible	Loving	Suspicious

Tender	Uncaring	Vital
Threatened	Ungrateful	Vulnerable
Tolerant	Unhelpful	Worried
Trusting	Unreserved	
Unafraid	Violent	

Choose several emotions and their opposites that describe the states and sensations you are or have been experiencing. Record them in your journal.

Practice 18: Welcoming Opposites of Feeling and Emotion

The following practice addresses opposites of emotion. You can do this same practice addressing opposites of feeling as well.

With your eyes open or closed, welcome the environment and sounds around you...the touch of air on your skin...the sensations where your body touches the surface that's supporting it...the feeling of your body breathing itself...sensations that are present throughout your body....

Now, welcome an emotion that's present in your body...or recall an emotion that you're working with in your life.... If no emotion is present, be with what's most calling your attention right now...and remember...you can always return to the safe haven of your inner resource whenever you feel the need to take a momentary time-out to feel secure and at ease....

And, if an emotion is present, where and how do you feel it in your body?... Are there thoughts or images that accompany this emotion?... Welcome your experience just as it is, without judging or trying to change it....

And, if it's helpful, locate an opposite of this emotion.... Where and how do you experience this opposite in your body?... If it's helpful, recall a memory that invites this opposite of emotion more fully into your body....

109

When it feels right, move back and forth between these opposites, experiencing first one, then its opposite, at your own pace...sensing how each emotion impacts your body and mind....

Then, when you're ready, sense both emotions at the same time.... Experience how this impacts your entire body and mind....

Sense how you are the observer of all that's now present in your awareness...awake and aware of all that's present...sensations...thoughts...images.... Affirm to yourself, *I am aware and awake, practicing iRest and resting at ease, welcoming opposites of emotion and being with everything just as it is.*

When you're ready, take time to write down in your journal your reflections from doing this practice. Any actions you've discovered you need to take become intentions that you plan to follow through with in your daily life.

■ 🔊 Practice 19: Creating Continuums of Opposites of Feeling and Emotion

It's important that the practice of iRest supports your healing, and not the continuation of your PTSD. In order to keep the focus on your healing, it's helpful to create a list of *continuums of opposites*, which is a series of paired opposites that relates to and describes how a particular emotion or experience begins and gains strength. In this way, a series of paired opposites describes a timeline of a particular feeling or emotion. You create continuums of opposites in order to more fully welcome a particular emotion or experience without activating your PTSD symptoms. First, you do this by working with less intense feelings and emotions, so you can build your tolerance, strength, and ability to handle more intense feelings and emotions later.

In the examples of continuums of opposites that follow, the emotions—chosen by actual iRest participants—are enraged, numb, and joyful. Before entering into their practice of Welcoming Opposites of Feeling and Emotion, each participant identified a series of pairs of opposites related to his or her emotional experience that he or she then worked with during the actual iRest practice.

During iRest, each pair of opposites is worked with step-by-step, feeling-by-feeling, or emotion-by-emotion until the entire continuum has been fully explored. Generally, this occurs during several iRest practices.

Read through the following examples. Notice how the pairs of opposites are related. Also, notice how the pairs of opposites describe the timeline of the emotion from its more subtle beginning to its intense end.

Enraged

Hot/Cool → *Edgy/Calm* → *Cranky/Peaceful* → *Irritable/Relaxed* → *Frustrated/At ease* → *Angry/Peaceful* → *Livid/Unperturbed* → *Furious/Unruffled* → *Enraged/Tranquil*

Numb

Cold/Warm → *Heartbeat fluttering/Heartbeat steady* → *Anxious/ Calm* → *Fearful/Courageous* → *Terrified/Brave* → *Paralyzed/ Responsive* → *Helpless/Engaged* → *Numb/Thriving*

Joyful

Warm/Cool → *Comfortable/Uncomfortable* → *Relaxed/Uneasy* → *Smiling/Frowning* → *Pleasurable/Painful* → *Happy/Sad* → *Glowing/ Contracted* → *Joyful/Miserable*

Now it's your turn. Choose an emotion you want to work with. Now, place your feelings and emotions in a series that forms a continuum. Write them down in your journal.

Once you've recorded a list of pairs of opposites in a continuum, write down each of the pairs on separate index cards. Arrange the pairs in the order that most accurately describes your emotion along a continuum. Keep or toss out pairs by following your instincts. Most people end up with four to six pairs of opposites for each continuum of emotion.

One way to achieve a timeline is to score each pair of opposites by assigning it a number on a scale from 1 to 100, with 100 being the highest level of the emotion imaginable and 1 being almost a complete absence of the emotion. Each pair takes its place in your continuum, according to its score of points. Write the score for each pair of opposites on the back of the index card. Give each pair the first score that pops into your head.

When each of your pairs of opposites has a score, sort your cards into a pile from 1 to 100. Use the table below to sort your pairs.

Intensity of Emotion	Score
Low Intensity	1–19
Medium–Low Intensity	20–39
Medium Intensity	40–59
Medium–High Intensity	60–79
High Intensity	80–100

The goal here is to end up with a pile of cards graded from 1 to 100. If this happens, congratulations! If not, go back and evaluate your pairs of opposite, or create new ones. When you're finished, combine all your cards into a pile that is ordered from lowest to highest intensity of emotion. This is your personal continuum for this particular emotion. Before your practice of the iRest tool Welcoming Opposites of Feeling and Emotion, take a moment to reflect on each pair of opposites.

Practice 20: Interweaving Your Inner Resource

It's helpful to affirm and interweave your inner resource (chapter 4) through every step you take during your practice of iRest. This helps you stay grounded and connected to yourself through even your most challenging feelings and emotions. Here's how to affirm and interweave your inner resource of well-being when you're engaging a particular feeling and emotion, or working with continuums of opposites.

With your eyes open or closed, welcome the environment and sounds around you...the touch of air on your skin...the sensations where your body touches the surface that's supporting it...the feeling of your body breathing itself...sensations that are present throughout your body....

Now, welcome and experience your inner resource within your body...your felt-sense of being secure...at ease...connected...grounded.... Take a few moments to welcome and experience your inner resource throughout your entire body....

Now, welcome in the feeling or emotion you're working with.... Now, again, feel your inner resource.... Now, again, experience the feeling and emotion.... Taking your time, feel, in turn, each opposite of feeling and emotion on your continuum, alternating with your inner resource of well-being.... Then, when you're ready, and at the same time, feel both your inner resource and both opposites of feeling and emotion.... Feel how this affects your body and mind. It's not possible to experience both opposites and your inner resource at the same time with your mind.... Instead of using your mind, sense with your body.... In order to feel everything together, allow your mind to defocus, and allow both opposites and your inner resource to all be present at the same time....

When you've completed this practice, take time to write down your reflections. Record actions you've discovered as intentions that you plan to follow through with in your daily life.

Remember the focusing and defocusing networks I talked about earlier in this chapter? When you attend to either of your opposites of feeling and emotion, you're activating the focusing network within your brain. When you experience your inner resource, or hold opposites at the same time as your inner resource, you're activating your defocusing network. When your defocusing network is activated, you're changing old, negative patterns.

You can practice interweaving your inner resource during specific practices of iRest or when you're beginning to experience a negative feeling or emotion. Interweaving your inner resource into all your life experiences helps you stay grounded and empowered, no matter where you are, who you're with, or what you're experiencing.

Putting It All Together

Now let's combine all of the practices involving feelings and emotions that we learned in this chapter into one practice.

Practice 21: Welcoming Feelings and Emotions

Set aside 30 to 40 minutes to experience this practice in a setting where you won't be disturbed.

Allow your senses to open to the environment and sounds around you... the sensation of air on your skin...the sensations where your body touches

the surface that's supporting you…. Scan your body and release any unnecessary tension…. Relax and let go into being at ease throughout your entire
body and mind….

Inner Resource

Bring your attention to your body and welcome your inner resource…your
felt-sense of well-being…ease…security…and feeling grounded….

Welcoming Feelings

Allow your attention to wander through your body…. Be aware of and
welcome feelings that are present…perhaps the feeling of warmth or coolness…heaviness or lightness…comfort or discomfort…feelings of tension
and of being at ease…without changing anything…simply welcoming feelings that are present just as they are….

Remember that you can always return to the safe haven of your inner
resource whenever you feel the need to take a momentary time-out to feel
grounded, secure, and at ease….

Locate and move between opposite feelings…. If you're sensing warmth,
find coolness…if heaviness, sense lightness…if comfort, then discomfort…
if tension, then ease…. Without going into thinking…just experience the
feeling that's currently present…. Then, come back to the original feeling…
then feel its opposite again…moving back and forth between opposites at
your own pace….

Then perceive both opposites at the same time…. Experience how per-
ceiving opposites at the same time acts on your entire body and mind…not
with the thinking mind…just sensing…just experiencing….

Now move between feeling your inner resource and experiencing opposites of feeling….

Feel your inner resource…then an opposite of feeling…then feel your
inner resource…then the other opposite of feeling…. Move from one experience to the other…inner resource…feeling…inner resource…feeling….

Now experience everything simultaneously…your inner resource and
both opposites of feeling…. Feel how this affects your body and your mind….

Welcoming Emotion

Now welcome an emotion that's present in your body…or recall a specific
emotion that you'd like to work with in this moment…. If it's helpful, recall

a memory that invites this emotion more fully into your body.... And if no emotion is present, this, too, is your experience, everything just as it is.... Be with what's most calling your attention right now...whether an emotion, a feeling, or another sensation....

Remember that you can always return to the safe haven of your inner resource whenever you feel the need to take a momentary time-out...to feel grounded, secure, and at ease....

And, if an emotion is present, where in your body do you feel it?... Are there thoughts or images that accompany this emotion?... Welcome your experience just as it is without judging it or trying to change it....

While sensing this emotion in your body, imagine a door opening and your emotion walking into your awareness.... What does your emotion look like?... What's its form?... Does it have a shape or is it shapeless?... Is it an animal, plant, mineral, or person?... Welcome your experience just as it is, however it is.... Invite it to stand or sit down at a comfortable distance from you and ask it, "What do you want?... Want do you need?... What action are you asking that I take in the world?"... With each question you ask, imagine yourself as the emotion speaking its answer back to you.... Take time now to ask these questions and hear the responses....

Now, locate an opposite emotion and where you experience this opposite in your body.... If it's helpful, recall a memory that invites this opposite of emotion more fully into your body....

Then, move back and forth between these opposites, experiencing first one, then its opposite, in your own rhythm.... Sense how each emotion affects your body and mind....

Then, sense both emotions simultaneously.... Sense how this acts on your entire body and mind....

Now, move between experiencing your inner resource and experiencing opposites of emotion...inner resource...then, first one emotion...then its opposite...moving from one experience to the other.... Now experience everything at the same time...inner resource and both opposites of emotion.... Feel how this affects your body and mind....

Completion

When you're ready, in your own rhythm and timing, gently open and close your eyes several times.... Bring your attention to your surroundings while sensing deep relaxation, ease, well-being, and peace throughout your body.... Affirm to yourself that as you go about your daily life—talking, walking, eating, working, playing, and even sleeping—sensations of deep relaxation and well-being are accompanying you in every moment.

At your leisure, and when you're ready, come fully back to your eyes-open state of wakefulness.... Be grateful for taking this time for yourself, for health, healing, and your practice of iRest....

When you're ready, take time to write in your journal about what you've just experienced. Note actions that you wish to carry out in your life. Write them down as intentions that support your heartfelt mission.

Moving Forward

The practices offered to you in this chapter teach you that your feelings and emotions are messengers. They're here to deliver important information to you about what it is you want, what it is you need, and what actions you need to take to empower you in your relationships and life.

Learning to respond to—rather than avoid, deny, or react to—your feelings and emotions is an important step in healing your PTSD. It entails listening and responding to the information that each feeling and emotion is delivering to you.

Just as it takes time to strengthen a muscle when working at the gym, it takes time to strengthen your ability to welcome and respond to your feelings and emotions. So take your time. Remember that you're following in the footsteps of thousands of others who have successfully learned how to respond to their feelings and emotions, and who have healed their PTSD. Let your footsteps be here, too, for others who follow behind you.

Chapter 8

Welcoming Opposites of Thought

Since I started practicing iRest, I realize that I have the ability to shift my negative thoughts into positive ones, which is helping me feel more in control of my life. I call this a miracle.

—Gulf War veteran

Feelings and emotions are the messengers sent to you by your body. *Cognitions*—which are made up of your thoughts, beliefs, images, and memories—are the messengers sent to you by your mind. We have an estimated 12,000 to 50,000 thoughts per day. These thoughts typically occur in a normal range from positive to neutral to negative and back again. PTSD causes hyperactivity in your mind, which upsets the normal range of your thoughts, causing an increase in negative thoughts. When you don't understand the role of both your positive and negative thoughts, you can feel out of control in your life and relationships. By welcoming and understanding both your positive and negative thoughts as messengers, you can engage new patterns of thinking that help you feel in control. In this chapter, you'll learn the role your thoughts play as messengers. You'll also learn how to use them to heal your PTSD.

Change Your Thoughts, Change Your Life

Your thinking mind is an amazing organ. It's the product of millions of years of evolution. Every day, you experience a wide range of thoughts—from positive and caring to negative and hurtful. You experience thoughts, images, and memories that create hope and connection, as well as ones that invite doubt and fear. Thoughts enable you to believe that you're powerful and capable of great things or that you're helpless and so limited that you'll never amount to anything at all. You see, what you think about yourself has tremendous power. In the words of Henry Ford, the founder of Ford Motor Company, "Whether you think you can, or you think you can't—you're right."

Every thought you have—whether it's *I'm capable of great things* or *I'm helpless*—impacts your body. As you read these words your thyroid, spleen, pancreas, and adrenal glands are responding to your thoughts by sending out hormones that are influencing your immune, cardiovascular, respiratory, and digestive systems. Like it or not, every thought you have has a powerful effect on your body, and every way that your body is feeling has a powerful effect on your thoughts (Dispenza 2012). Now, relate this understanding to your PTSD. Your negative thoughts affect your body and hold you captive in your PTSD. In turn, your bodily symptoms of PTSD hold you captive in your thoughts. Your negative thoughts create a vicious cycle that keeps your PTSD in place.

Change your thinking, and you change your PTSD. How? Change your thinking, and you change your body. Change your body, and you change how you feel. Change how you feel, and you change your thinking. Change your thinking in this moment, and you change how you think and feel in the next moment. Change how you think and feel in the next moment, and you change how you think and feel for the rest of your life (Dispenza 2012; Graham 2013; Hanson 2013, 2009). You gain the power to heal your PTSD when you understand that, with a single thought, you can change your life. *If you think you can, you can.*

You Can't Outrun a Thought

Working with thoughts is a lot like encountering a bear in the wild. If you run from your thoughts, your thoughts will chase you. You can't outrun a bear. Nor can you outrun your thoughts. Being prepared for encounters with negative thoughts is your best way of surviving thought attacks (Boykin 1998). iRest tool #7, Welcoming Opposites of Thought, teaches you skills to survive thought attacks. Just as a safety program for hikers prepares you to deal with bears in the wild, the iRest program prepares you to deal with thoughts, beliefs, images, and memories in your daily life.

Using Welcoming Opposites of Thought when you encounter a negative or intense thought enables you to:

- Stop and sense the thought you're having.

- Stay calm.

- Face the thought.

- Speak with authority.

- Let the thought know you mean it no harm.

- See what the thought wants.

- Take appropriate action.

iRest teaches you to not run from but face your thoughts. It teaches you how to stay calm and stand up to your thoughts with gentle firmness. Remember that every thought is a messenger. Your thoughts are here to give you information for how to respond and proceed in your life. Welcoming Opposites of Thought teaches you how to relate to every thought as a messenger so that you can enjoy, respond, and use your thoughts to thrive in your life.

The Life Cycle of a Thought

Thoughts are constantly changing. As thoughts change, they go through five stages: birth, growth, stability, decay, and death. Every thought you have is born and will die.

When you identify with negative thoughts that arise because of your PTSD, you may take these thoughts to be your only truth. When you do that, you become stuck in the mud of your negative thought patterns. When you get stuck in negative thought patterns, these thoughts will keep recurring. They will keep trying to get your attention. It may feel like you'll never be able to change recurring negative thoughts, such as, *I'm broken, I'm helpless, I'm not enough,* and *I should have done it differently.* But, in actuality, thoughts do change. Remember, just like feelings and emotions, your negative thoughts are messengers. They're trying to show you the positive actions you can take to restore health and harmony in your life. When you face your thoughts, when you recognize what they want and take the actions they request, you break your negative thought cycles and climb out of the mud of your thoughts. When you truly hear the underlying positive messages your thoughts carry, you release them to go on to complete their stages of life. They'll pass away and disappear, for they've served their purpose. Your thoughts can change. Your PTSD can change.

iRest Tool #7: Welcoming Opposites of Thought

This iRest tool teaches you how to become aware of and *dis-identify* from your negative thoughts. This tool teaches you to break your connection to your harmful thoughts, beliefs, images, and memories.

An important skill for healing PTSD is your ability to experience opposites of your negative thoughts. Every thought you have arrives paired with its opposite. *I'm broken* cannot exist without *I'm whole. I'm powerless* cannot exist without *I'm capable. I'm not enough* cannot exist without *I'm enough. I should have done it differently* can't exist without the opposite *I did the best I knew how.*

Pairs of opposites are like two sides of a coin. When you believe only one-half of a pair of opposites is true, such as *I'm helpless,* you become stuck in that belief. When you become stuck in a one-sided belief, suffering and conflict arise. The good news is that your feeling of being stuck, as well as your sense of suffering and conflict, all arrive as messengers to tell you that you've become stuck in a belief and in one side of your experience. Healing begins when you realize that the feeling of being stuck is a messenger that wants you to recognize and consider its opposite.

Through the iRest practice of Welcoming Opposites of Thought, you learn to experience both sides of the coin. This enables you to dis-identify from your mistaken beliefs. Healing your PTSD takes place when you open to the full experience of both sides of the coin.

The Trap of the Shoulds

Your attempt to get rid of one-half of a pair of opposites only creates conflict. Trying to live your life only feeling *I'm capable* without a willingness to feel *I'm helpless* begins and ends in conflict. That way of living is based on the belief that only one-half of this pair of opposites *should* be true. You believe that you should always feel "capable" and never "helpless." Only when you welcome every opposite of life—helpless and capable, shameful and powerful, sadness and happiness, fear and safety—are you able to go beyond these pairs of opposites and find true healing, health, and freedom.

Your mind is biologically programmed to identify with whatever thought or belief is present. That's its nature. One of the primary thoughts your mind identifies with is, *I should have* _____ . This thought reveals your mind's tendency to identify with only one-half of a pair of opposites—the negative half. This tendency is part of your mind's *negativity bias,* or your preference to perceive the negative more readily than the positive (see chapter 4).

When you identify with the thought *I should have...,* you can get caught in a *trap of shoulds.* Here, your belief of how you *should be* holds you hostage in conflict and suffering. For example, holding on to *I should have done more* prevents you from understanding *I did the best I knew how. I should have done more* prevents you from accepting that you were actually powerless to do anything other than what you did do in the moment. To release yourself from this trap, you need to take time to feel and experience the opposite of your shoulds. When you have the whole experience and picture, you take informed actions that move you forward into your life and healing.

Pairing Opposites Promotes Healing

During the iRest practice of Welcoming Opposites of Thought, negative thoughts, beliefs, memories, and images are paired with their opposites. This practice of pairing opposites builds your tolerance for experiencing both negative *and* positive thoughts as they arise in your daily life. iRest teaches you to welcome all opposites rather than resist them, especially the ones you call "negative." When you understand that all thoughts are messengers, you realize that they are neither "good" nor "bad." They just "are." Thoughts are messengers here to help you heal.

As you learn to welcome your thoughts as messengers, psychological integration and healing takes place. Psychological integration and healing builds your capacity to embrace the changing and troublesome circumstances of your life. As you strengthen your ability to hold opposites, you also strengthen your ability to dis-identify and become free from being held hostage by one side of a pair of opposites. Dis-identification frees you to recognize the empowering actions you need to take to deal with any negative or positive thought or situation that arises. Welcoming opposites enables you to experience a calmness and peace within yourself that cannot be ruffled by any thought, belief, image, or memory. Then, you're able to fully experience and enjoy the qualities of well-being, joy, love, compassion, and peace in your life and relationships.

Step Back and Gain Perspective

Your thoughts are "objects" that you can be aware of. Like any object, then, it's possible for you to step back from your thoughts and view them from a distance. Stepping back enables you to get a better view of them and any related situation. From this improved perspective, you're more able to see and understand the actions you need to take.

Tom, who grew up experiencing repeated psychological and physical trauma in his household, reports that when he takes a moment to step back from his negative thoughts, he imagines himself in a helicopter flying around his thoughts and viewing them from various angles. He's come to realize, through his practice of iRest, that he's not doomed to remain connected with his negative thoughts for the rest of his life. As he "flies" around his thoughts, he learns to invite himself to consider their opposites. Tom reports that this newfound ability brings him a sense of relief that he'd neither known nor experienced before engaging this iRest practice of stepping back, gaining perspective, and welcoming opposites.

Like Tom, you can learn to step back, gain perspective, and welcome the opposites of the negative thoughts, beliefs, memories, and images that hold you hostage. When you're caught in a cycle of harmful thoughts, you tend to lose track of your inner wisdom and guidance. Rather than seeing your negative thoughts as helpful messengers, you tend to see them as aggressive bears and run from them. When you refuse to face your thoughts, over time you no longer hear their voices as requests for your attention. You only hear them screaming at you. When this occurs, you fall into the trap of believing that your negative thoughts are something you need to escape. It's important that you learn to interact with your thoughts as messengers, which are wanting your attention to help you heal your PTSD.

> *Stuart, a Gulf War vet, became lost in the thought "I'm helpless" after a mission during which his best friend was killed in front of him in a roadside explosion. Stuart was left feeling "helpless" because he believed that "I should have been able to do something to save my friend." Over time, because Stuart never stopped to welcome his feeling of "I'm helpless" and his belief that "I should have been able to do something," his feeling and belief fused together. This fusion of feeling and belief created a negative spiral inside of Stuart's mind that degraded into feelings of guilt and shame in his body. The sense of helplessness so tormented Stuart that when he returned home from his tour of duty, he began to believe that he was helpless in the rest of his life.*
>
> *During iRest, Stuart was invited to "step back" and relate to his feelings and beliefs as messengers that were trying to get his attention. He learned that he was no longer hearing the real message that they were trying to deliver. As he learned to step back and consider the opposites of his feelings and beliefs, he realized that, in the moment of his friend's death, there was nothing he could have done other than what he did. He was helpless in that moment. When he was invited to consider*

actions that might empower him, Stuart imagined a conversation with his friend that helped him resolve his feelings of guilt and loss. This conversation allowed him to move on with his life. Through iRest, Stuart realized that whenever he feels that he's being held hostage by his feelings and thoughts, it's time for him to welcome them in as messengers. He's learning that his thoughts and feelings are here to help him find the right course of action for every situation in his life.

iRest teaches you how to relate to your thoughts as messengers, so you can truly welcome and accept their messages. Your actions of welcoming and accepting the messages from your thoughts empower you to uncover the actions you need to take to move fully into your life and relationships. Relate to all your thoughts as messengers, and you have a powerful tool in your tool belt for healing PTSD.

Thoughts Have Feelings

How do you know you're having a particular thought or belief? You know because every thought gives rise to particular sensations, which you experience in your body as feelings or emotions. For example, when you believe *I'm broken,* or the opposite, *I'm okay as I am,* you feel a certain way in your body. Your heart contracts or opens. Your gut tightens or relaxes. You feel sad and depressed, or happy and peaceful. Bodysensing and breathsensing are iRest tools that help you notice and experience the sensations, feelings, and emotions that are associated with each thought you have. The iRest tools that teach you to welcome opposites of feelings, emotions, and thoughts show you how to work with your thoughts, sensations, feelings, and emotions so that you can heal your PTSD and feel empowered in your relationships and life.

As you practice the following exercise, take time to register the thought, belief, image, or memory that you're working with, as well as the sensations, feelings, and emotions that come along with it. In order to heal PTSD, you need to learn how to notice your thoughts, beliefs, memories, and images, as well as to feel where and how each one affects your body and mind.

Practice 22: Welcoming Opposites of Thought

With your eyes gently open or closed, take a moment to ease back in the position you're in and welcome the environment and sounds around you… the touch of air on your skin…the sensations where your body touches the surface that's supporting it…the feeling of your body breathing itself…sensations that are present throughout your body…thoughts that are present in your mind….

Locate a recurring negative thought that you associate with your PTSD. Or take one of the negative thoughts I've previously mentioned, such as *I'm broken, I'm powerless, I'm not enough,* or *I should have done it differently.* In your journal, write down the thought you want to welcome.

Affirm this thought as your only truth and reality…. When you take this thought to be true, where and how do you feel it in your body?… Do you feel it in your gut, heart, or throat?… Do you feel relaxed or tense, opened up or closed down?… How do you act or react in your life and relationships when you believe that this thought about yourself is true?… Take a few moments and write down words that describe how you feel when you take this thought to be true.

Now turn your attention to imagining an opposite thought…. For instance, *I'm broken* becomes *I'm whole. I'm powerless* becomes *I'm capable. I'm not enough* becomes *I'm okay just as I am. I should have done it differently* becomes *I did it the best I knew how.* Welcome this opposite thought and write it down.

Affirm this opposite thought as your only truth and reality…. When you take this opposite thought to be true, where and how do you feel it in your body?… Do you feel it in your gut, heart, or throat?… Do you feel relaxed or tense, opened up or closed down?… How do you react when you believe that this opposite thought is true?… Take a few moments and write down how you feel when you take this thought to be true.

Now, experience both opposites at the same time…. First, affirm and experience in your body your negative thought; for example, *I'm helpless.* Then, experience in your body the opposite; that is, *I'm capable,* et cetera… first one, then the other…. Take your time…. Go back and forth, affirming each opposite thought while also experiencing how and where each impacts your body…. After several rounds of going back and forth, experiencing each opposite in turn, affirm and experience both thoughts at the same time….

A hint here: Don't affirm your beliefs with only your thinking mind.... Your task is to feel and experience both thoughts at the same time along with the effects that they have on your body.... Don't try to merge opposites into one another.... Experience both opposites at the same time and allow whatever happens to happen. Holding opposites of thoughts at the same time is a creative moment that takes you beyond either opposite into a world of new and infinite possibilities.

Take a few moments and write down in your journal your reflections on this practice. Are there any actions that you wish to take as a result of the practice? Are there any intentions that come out of this practice? How do these intentions support your heartfelt mission?

Here's what Rebecca discovered when she was invited to consider opposites of the belief she was carrying inside herself:

Rebecca felt traumatized by the three rounds of chemotherapy she'd endured in dealing with colon cancer. She came to me for an iRest session with the intention of learning how to find relief from the racing thoughts she was experiencing in response to having cancer. Rebecca let me know that there was a particular belief she wanted to work with during iRest. She said, "I feel that I'm a failure. I'm a nutritionist and healer, and while I've helped countless others, I've been unable to affect the course of my own cancer treatment." As we talked, Rebecca stated her core belief as "I'm a failure and I'm unlovable," and its opposite as "I'm lovable. I do the best I can."

When Rebecca reflected on her belief I'm a failure and I'm unlovable, she felt sad and began to cry. When she reflected on the belief I'm lovable and I do the best I can, she felt uplifted. When Rebecca experienced both beliefs at the same time, her face began to glow, as she realized that both these beliefs were part of a larger wholeness. She said, "When I hold them at the same time, I realize that, actually, I'm love itself, and that I'm always doing the best I know how. If I'm love itself, I can tolerate being unloved and failing at times." This realization had a deep and lasting effect on Rebecca's life.

In the following weeks, Rebecca took time each day to experience and deeply feel I'm love, itself. I'm always doing the best I know how. As a result, she was able to let go of her belief I'm a failure and unlovable. She reported feeling a deep sense of intimacy with others and herself. She said, "I'm no longer looking to people for love and wholeness—I found love and wholeness within myself."

You Are Wholeness

During iRest, you learn to welcome every experience you have as an aspect of your *wholeness*. Your mind may resist this understanding by exclaiming, *How could this thought, this belief, this image, this memory be an aspect of wholeness?* That thought is doubt entering as another messenger. Doubt is one of the many thoughts you experience that leads your mind to divide what's *whole* into separate pieces. Remember, every *thing* arises with its opposite. Opposites are never separate. They are two parts that come together in a field of wholeness. When any sensation, emotion, or thought arises, its opposite always arises along with it. Neither is separate from the other. And neither is separate from the field of wholeness. When you welcome and hold opposites at the same time, you can have a glimpse, just as Rebecca did, of the greater wholeness from which you and your thoughts arise. The iRest program, with its powerful focus on welcoming opposites, is based on the insight that by healing the root belief of separation, you're able to heal PTSD and find true and lasting peace in your life.

I have witnessed countless people in the depths of despair suddenly become joyful, even as they continue to experience grief. Your mind may view opposites such as grief and joy, anger and peace, and shame and confidence as mismatched. Ultimately, as true healing unfolds, all opposites are seen as two complementary parts that arise within a field of wholeness. As iRest reveals your wholeness (see chapter 11), you realize that you don't have to change your circumstance to experience health, healing, and peace. As you accept what life brings to you just as it is, you're able to welcome the opposites of your everyday life and find true peace of mind.

Moving Forward

In the coming chapters, you'll learn practices that help you expand your ability to welcome opposites so that you can truly experience your wholeness of being. Experiencing your wholeness reveals the essential essence of yourself that can never be harmed by trauma and PTSD. As you learn to welcome opposites, and experience your wholeness, you increase your ability to experience deep relaxation. You also open the doorway to experiencing an expansive feeling of joy that is independent of your circumstance. So let us turn our attention to iRest tool #8: Welcoming Joy and Well-Being!

Chapter 9

Welcoming Joy and Well-Being

iRest helps me feel light again. I used to feel like this a long time ago. But then the flashbacks came, and I silenced them with drugs. Darkness consumed my life with my wife and kids, and in my job. Through practicing iRest, I've realized that choosing darkness is my choice. So, I said to myself, *I can choose light instead*. Now, when the feeling that causes me to choose darkness comes, I do iRest. iRest helps me choose light. Now I know that change is in my hands. Before, I didn't have a tool of my own to deal with the flashbacks. Now I do. I'm smiling much more and feeling more at ease with myself.

—Vietnam vet

You may believe that joy comes to you when you have what you want. You may believe that when you have a good job, enough money, an attentive lover, healthy food, and a peaceful home, you'll have joy. Similarly, when you're experiencing what you don't want—depression, grief, pain, loss, or PTSD—you may believe joy is absent. You're not alone in this belief. I, too, was taught that the experience of joy depends on having some desired object or circumstance. Even the Merriam-Webster dictionary defines joy as dependent on achieving "well-being, success, or good fortune, or by the prospect of possessing what one desires." It's no wonder joy has gotten confused with desire and achievement.

I've come to understand joy differently. Through the practice of iRest, I've learned that true joy is not connected to desire or achievement. I've discovered that there are, in fact, two types of joy:

1. Joy that comes with an achievement

2. Joy that exists independent of whatever else is present

In this chapter, I'll discuss the role of joy in healing your PTSD and teach you how to cultivate joy in every moment of your daily life. Welcome joy!

Joy Just Is

The practice of iRest will not create joy. Joy is already inside you, waiting to be released. Joy exists independently from your PTSD and any other state of your mind or body. Joy exists without a reason. Joy just is. Like your ability to learn a language or to love another human being, joy is a natural capacity that's yours at birth (Baraz and Alexander 2010). That joy is your birthright explains why, even in the midst of pain and suffering, loss and grief, sadness and depression, you can still feel joy. Joy is always present, waiting to be experienced in the midst of what is, no matter what is.

I understand that experiencing joy, along with the symptoms of your PTSD and other struggles, can challenge your way of thinking. It's important that you understand that when you resist or deny joy, you lessen the importance of your life, as well as the lives of those around you (Gilbert 2007). You can survive with or without objects, pleasures, or achievements. In order to thrive, however, you need joy. Your ability to experience joy is directly related to your ability to fully live your life and appreciate the lives of others. The practice of iRest can help you welcome joy in your life no matter what else you may be experiencing. Because true joy exists independent of pain and suffering, it offers you a gateway for healing PTSD.

Here is Jan's experience of unexpectedly discovering joy in the midst of the pain of her PTSD:

I'm constantly upset with the people around me and with myself. I have a really hard time dealing with everyday pressures. Struggle is the norm of my daily life. My last iRest session changed that. It was incredible. First, I was practicing welcoming my anger, and then I welcomed its opposite, relaxation. From there, I moved on to welcoming both opposites. As I was doing that, my mind suddenly cried out, So this is the joy of being! *The experience was one of deep and profound joy. From head to toe, joy coursed through my body. A great sense of relaxation and calmness came over my mind. The incredible thing was that I realized I've known this joy all my life. I'd just ignored it while I paid more attention to my anger and upset. I never knew I could feel joy in the midst of being upset. This is going to make a big difference in how I deal with myself and others in the future.*

The Joy of Being

Joy comes in many flavors. For some, it's a feeling of well-being. For others, it's a feeling of contentment, enthusiasm, radiance, or connection—or the feeling of simply being (Baraz and Alexander 2010).

In chapter 3, I introduced you to the felt-sense of being. When you're able to rest in and as being, you discover your birthright of well-being, contentment, and joy. Here are some of the words others have used to describe their experience of being: *indescribable yet undeniable…peaceful …calm…open…everywhere, yet nowhere specific…warm…heart-centered… presence…loving…safe…calm…connected…refuge…sanctuary…well-being….* Another word that people use to describe being is *joy.*

The search for joy motivates much of what you do in your life. However, it is your search for a lasting joy that can prevent you from feeling the underlying joy of being. Searching keeps your mind fixed on external objects and experiences. Looking for joy maintains your belief that joy is dependent on getting a certain object or having a specific experience. Looking for something outside yourself takes you away from seeing that joy is already present within you. It's waiting to be seen, felt, and expressed. Here is Ken's description of realizing joy:

Before coming to the practice of iRest, I'd read hundreds of books. I'd worked with several therapists, studied with various teachers, and tried everything from drugs to meditation to end my depression and find peace. Then, during one iRest practice, I heard the two words just be. I'd never thought of that before. It was so simple. I was astonished when I realized I could just be. By just being, I could feel joy in the midst of my depression. No one had ever told me that before. Since discovering joy inside of me, I'm more able to be with my depression. iRest is helping me be with myself in ways I'd never considered before coming to this practice.

Joy Is Good Medicine

Since ancient times, joy has been recognized as a powerful healing force. For example, in early Greece, hospitals were built near amphitheaters so patients could easily attend comedies that doctors prescribed to promote healing (Sesana 2013). "Laughter is the best medicine," the familiar adage derived from a biblical proverb, is another example that points to our understanding of joy as good medicine. Today's research, including studies on the effects of meditation practices, such as iRest, confirms the healing power of joy (Lemonick 2005).

Studies show that regularly experiencing joy produces healthy changes throughout your body, brain, and nervous system. Specifically, the effects of joy have been shown to strengthen your immune system, boost your energy, diminish pain, and protect you from the damaging effects of stress. This means that cultivating joy in your life improves your resistance to disease. Also—most important to healing your PTSD—joy has a positive effect on reducing cortisol levels in your body. Remember cortisol? It is the stress hormone associated with PTSD. When PTSD symptoms go on for long periods of time, your body's production of cortisol increases, which thereby decreases the healthy function of your immune system (Fried et al. 1998). Joy is the perfect antidote to keep cortisol production in balance. And joy is the perfect "medicine" for strengthening your immune system (Berk and Tan 1995; Berk, Tan, and Fry 1993; Berk, Tan, Fry et al. 1989; Berk, Tan, Napier et al. 1989; Berk et al. 1988).

Joy and well-being aren't just vague feelings; they are physical states of your body and brain that you can actively experience through meditation

(Lemonick 2005). Joy promotes your overall sense of well-being by activating your natural healing processes and releasing feel-good chemicals throughout your body (Graham 2013). The best thing about joy is that it has only positive effects (Berk and Tan 1995; Berk, Tan, and Fry 1993; Berk, Tan, Fry et al. 1989; Berk, Tan, Napier et al. 1989; Berk et al. 1988).

We all know moments of joy, and we all know how joy raises our spirits, even if these moments are few and far between. So the next time you find yourself experiencing joy at any level, know that you're doing good for your body, mind, health, and PTSD. Joy *is* good medicine.

Enhancing Joy by Vaccinating Against Stress

It's true that regularly experiencing joy helps reduce stress and heal PTSD. It's also true that regularly experiencing mild to moderate doses of negative emotions and thoughts is beneficial to your health, healing, and well-being. Why is this so? Research shows that your willingness to regularly experience mild to moderate stress and negative emotions builds your ability to bounce back from unpleasant situations (Rodriguez 2013; Pennebaker and Chung 2007; Pennebaker 2001). This means your willingness to welcome lower levels of stress helps protect you from being overwhelmed by higher levels of stress. Building your tolerance for mild to moderate stress makes more room for you to experience joy in your life. Just like those childhood vaccines that protected you from measles and polio, experiencing low levels of stress, as well as regularly experiencing joy, will vaccinate you against being overwhelmed by higher levels of stress.

Practice 23: Enhancing Joy

Here's a practice of iRest that can help enhance your experience of joy through your willingness to experience moderate doses of stress. iRest invites you to treat each stressful life event you encounter as an opportunity to vaccinate yourself against stress and strengthen your ability to welcome and experience joy. You can seize this opportunity in any moment. Try it now!

With your eyes gently open or closed, welcome the environment and sounds around you...the touch of air on your skin...the sensations where your body touches the surface that's supporting it...your body breathing...the various sensations that are present throughout your body....

Now, locate the felt-sense of joy in your body.... You may feel joy in any number of ways: as the feeling of connection, well-being, contentment, peace, enthusiasm, or some other sensation particular to your body and mind.... As you locate the felt-sense of joy in your body, sense where and how you experience it.... Perhaps it's a warm feeling in your heart...or a gentle smile on your face...or a glow in your belly that radiates out to your arms and legs.... Welcome the feeling of joy, however you experience it in your body and mind.... If it's helpful, bring to mind a memory of a person, animal, place, or object that brings a sense of joy into your body.... Allow the feeling of joy to grow and spread throughout your body....

Now, pair the feeling of joy with a negative sensation, emotion, or thought, or with a stressor you're experiencing.... Whether a situation, image, or memory...feel how this stressful thought, emotion, or situation affects your body and mind....

Now, alternate between experiencing the felt-sense of joy and the negative stressor.... Go back and forth, alternating by first feeling joy in your body, then the negative stressor in your body....

Now, take time to feel both at the same time...joy and stress...joy and the negative stressor.... Allow joy to spread throughout your body even as you're feeling the negative stress....

Then, when it feels right, let go of the negative stressor and come back to just feeling joy spreading throughout your body and mind.... Rest here for as long as you feel comfortable....

When you're ready to complete this practice, let your eyes open and close several times as you welcome the felt-sense of joy to accompany you in your daily activities and life....

Try this practice the next time you're experiencing a negative sensation, emotion, thought, image, or memory. You'll be surprised by how this simple exercise can have such a life-changing effect.

Go Easy on Yourself

It's only natural to evaluate your actions when you make a mistake. You want to understand what went wrong in order to avoid making the same mistake again. Sometimes the self-evaluations you make are fair and understanding. These are characteristics of a positive self-evaluation. Other times, your self-evaluations are unjust and unreasonable. These are the results of negative self-evaluations that are based in *self-criticism.*

You may believe that self-criticism will make you less likely to repeat your mistakes. I understand that you may feel this way, but I'm here to explain to you that negative self-criticism doesn't work.

Research shows that self-criticism doesn't motivate. Actually, it has been found to decrease motivation and future performance. On the other hand, honest self-evaluation, when coupled with self-compassion—being warm, kind, and supportive toward yourself—does work (Breines and Chen 2012). That's right. It's your ability to positively evaluate your actions that helps you grow from your mistakes and develop wisdom. When you're able to be honest with yourself without being critical, you build self-trust. Trusting yourself decreases anxiety, depression, and other symptoms of PTSD. The resulting peace of mind that comes from decreased symptoms of PTSD and increased self-trust inspires you to make the improvements you need to enhance your motivation and future performance (Hanson 2013; Breines and Chen 2012; Graham 2013; McGonigal 2012).

Now, let me give you a practical way to address self-criticism when it pops up in your life. The next time you feel self-critical, remember that self-criticism, like everything, is a messenger. Self-criticism is a part of your *negativity bias* (see chapter 4). When it arises, it can catch you off guard and lead to a chain of negative associations. Remember, though, that self-criticism arises along with its positive opposite, *self-compassion.* Welcome self-compassion along with self-criticism to grow your capacity to positively respond to yourself and your actions.

iRest Tool #8: Welcoming Joy and Well-Being

Now, let's put the welcoming of self-criticism and self-compassion into practice, so that you can fully experience their relationship to one another and to joy. Through this practice, you'll discover the actions that you can take to help you feel in harmony with yourself and the world around you. Whether you read or listen to a recording of the following practice, take time to pause along the way so that you can fully experience each part.

Practice 24: Welcoming Joy and Well-Being

Welcome the sounds around you...the sensation of air on your skin...the sensations of your body touching the surface that's supporting you.... Welcome your body breathing.... Welcome sensations in your body that are calling your attention....

Inner Resource

Welcome your inner resource...your felt-sense of well-being...ease...security...and feeling grounded.... Remember, you can always return to the comfort of your inner resource whenever you experience the need to feel grounded, secure, and at ease....

Emotions and Thoughts

Welcome emotions and thoughts that are calling your attention.... Sense where and how you feel them in your body and mind.... If it feels right, take a few moments now and interact with them by asking them what they want, what they need, and what actions they're asking you to take in your life.... Or just welcome and be with what's most calling your attention....

Welcoming Joy and Well-Being

Welcome an experience or memory of joy in whatever form it comes to you.... For example, the felt-sense of joy, peace, contentment, or well-being.... If it's helpful, recall a time or place when you were with a special friend, animal, object, or by yourself...a time or place that invites the feeling of joy.... If a memory comes into your awareness, enliven it with all your senses.... Recall tastes, smells, sounds, sights, feelings, thoughts, and images that you associate with your feeling of joy.... Allow joy to come fully into your body....

Allow joy to fill your torso...arms and legs...neck and head...your entire body experiencing joy.... Allow your entire body to fully welcome in this experience of joy....

Then, allow all thoughts, memories, and associations to dissolve, while you remain with the feeling of joy...joy independent of memory...joy independent of thinking.... Allow joy to spread throughout your entire body...joy throughout your entire body...joy filling every cell of your body....

Joy spreading throughout your body, and joy all around your body...with each exhalation and inhalation, feel joy growing...joy everywhere....

Be aware of the feeling of being, as well as the feeling of joy...simply being...and the feeling of joy.... Be aware of the various movements of sensation that are present...sensation...and joy...emotions...and joy...sounds... and joy...the feeling of the space around you...and joy...being and joy....

Integration

When it feels right, allow your eyes to open and close several times while continuing to experience the felt-sense of being and joy.... Allow yourself to come fully back to your wide-awake state of mind and body while continuing to feel joy and the felt-sense of simply being....

Before moving on, take a few minutes and record your reflections of this practice in your journal. Then, as you move back into your day, feel how being and joy are always present, no matter what else you may be experiencing.

Before going into the following practice, take a few minutes to write down or simply reflect on several events that you would describe as stressful in your life. Feel free to focus on either present or past events. Be sure to make note of the sensations, emotions, and thoughts that are associated with the stressful events. You'll use this information as you move through the following practice. To teach you how to welcome joy even when you're experiencing stress, you'll be invited to welcome each of the emotions, thoughts, and sensations along with your felt-sense of joy.

Practice 25: Welcoming Joy with Stress

Welcome the environment and sounds around you...the sensation of air where it touches your skin...the sensations of your body touching the surface that's supporting you...your body breathing...the various sensations that are calling your attention in your body....

Inner Resource

Welcome your inner resource...your sense of well-being...ease...security... and feeling grounded.... Remember, you can always return to the comfort of your inner resource whenever you experience the need to feel grounded, secure, and at ease....

Joy and Stress

Welcome the experience of joy in your body.... Take your time.... Allow the felt-sense of joy to come alive within your body and mind....

Now, recall one of the stressful events you reflected upon at the beginning of this practice.... Locate and experience the felt-sense of stress that this event brings into your body.... Whether it's a sensation, emotion, thought, or memory, feel where and how you experience this stress in your body and mind....

Now, go back and forth, several times...first experiencing the felt-sense of joy...then experiencing the stressful feeling...back and forth...at your own pace....

When it feels right, experience both joy and the stressful feeling at the same time...joy and the stressful sensation, emotion, thought, or memory.... Allow joy to be present at the same time as the felt-sense of stress.... Feel how this registers in your body and mind.... Take a few minutes now and continue doing this with each stressful event on your list....

When you feel complete in your work with your list and are ready to move on, allow any feelings of stress that remain to be just as they are.... Let go of thinking and fully welcome the experience of joy in your body...joy independent of memory...joy independent of stress.... Allow joy to expand fully...joy throughout your entire body...joy expanding to fill the space within, throughout, and all around your body.... With each exhalation and inhalation, feel joy growing...joy everywhere....

Feel joy everywhere...and the felt-sense of just being...feeling joy as a quality of being that's always present....

Be aware of sensations, emotions, and thoughts that are present.... Be aware of the feeling of joy and being that are also present.... Be aware of being, joy, and the various movements that are present...sensations and joy...emotions and joy...sounds and joy...the feeling of the space around you and joy...being and joy.... When it feels right, allow your eyes to open and close several times while continuing to feel joy and being....

Integration

When you feel ready, allow yourself to come fully back to your wide-awake state of body and mind while continuing to feel joy and the felt-sense of being.... Sense the world around you and the felt-sense of joy.... Sense the world around you and the felt-sense of being....

Before moving on, take a few minutes and record your reflections of this practice in your journal. Then, as you move back into your everyday life, feel how joy and being are always present, no matter what else you're experiencing.

Joy Invites Restful Sleep

Welcoming and experiencing joy reduces stress, increases well-being, boosts your immune system, reduces anxiety, decreases depression, and enhances your ability to sleep restfully through the night (Robotham, Chakkalackal, and Cyhlarova 2011; Seligman 2011, 2002). Getting restful sleep is directly related to healing your PTSD (Van Liempt 2012). After their first experience with iRest, participants often report that they're able to sleep through the night for the first time in months, even years. Here's what one Vietnam veteran wrote about his experience with iRest:

> *I'm a Vietnam veteran with PTSD. I think iRest is the best program I've had the pleasure to participate in. It's given me the first restful sleep I've had since Vietnam. When I'm having trouble falling asleep, I practice the tools I've learned in iRest. These tools help me get to sleep, stay asleep, and feel rested in the morning.*

Restoring your ability to get restful sleep is a positive side effect of practicing iRest. Through the iRest tools Practicing Bodysensing and Practicing Breathsensing, you learn to ease your body and mind into deep states of relaxation that support you to fall asleep, stay asleep, and get restful sleep. These practices—along with the iRest tools Affirming Your Inner Resource, Experiencing Being Awareness, and Experiencing Your Wholeness—enable you to shift your brain from its focusing network to its defocusing network (chapter 7). Doing this enables your body and mind to more easily enter into restful sleep patterns (Graham 2013).

iRest teaches you how to fall asleep, and how to go back to sleep. iRest "naps," daily practices of 8 to 12 minutes, can help you fall into short periods of restful sleep and awaken refreshed and ready for the rest of your day. Taking an iRest nap is one of the most effective tools to promote well-being and heal your PTSD (Mednick and Erhman 2006). Every night, you can use these iRest tools to help you fall asleep easily and quickly. If you wake in the middle of the night, you can use these same practices to help you fall asleep again. These practices have the power to bring your brain into the deep and restful sleep patterns necessary for healing all health concerns, including PTSD (Mednick and Erhman 2006; Miller 2013).

Paradoxical Sleep

The kind of rest you get during an iRest practice can be the same kind of rest you get during a deep sleep. But your sleep experience during iRest can sometimes feel unusual. Let me explain. At times, during iRest, you may hear your body snoring. In this case your body's asleep even though you experience yourself as awake. This experience is called *paradoxical sleep*. If you were in a sleep lab with electrodes attached to your head, your brain would be registering deep sleep waves, even though you feel yourself awake. During the practice of iRest, your body *is* getting the deep rest that it needs for healing and health.

At other times, when you're listening to the voice of someone leading you through the practice, you may no longer hear the words being spoken to you. You may later realize that, while practicing iRest, you fell into deep, restful sleep. At the end of your practice, you may wonder if you were doing the practice correctly, because you lost track of where you were in the practice or you fell asleep. Experiencing your body asleep and yourself awake, falling totally asleep, or coming back unsure about how you participated in the practice are all common experiences while practicing iRest. Rest assured that your practice is providing your body and mind with the rest you need for enhancing your health and healing your PTSD. Over the years, I've heard and read the testimonials of hundreds of people who say that even though they regularly fall asleep during the practice, or lose touch with the sound of my voice, they've found that their depression has cleared, their pain has lessened or disappeared, they're getting restful sleep at night, and their PTSD has diminished or cleared completely. Here's what one woman told me about falling asleep during iRest:

> *I'm usually a very angry person. I make myself and everyone around me uncomfortable. During my iRest sessions I usually*

fall asleep, so at first I didn't think anything would come from my doing this practice. But over these past weeks something's changed inside of me. I used to get upset and hit people and things, throw chairs, and kick walls. I'm not doing that anymore. I feel more centered. I find myself feeling a lot of joy during my days, and people are saying that they like being around me. I tend to have a lot of negative thoughts in my head. But now I find myself reflecting on things rather than reacting the way I used to. Stress and drama seem to be falling out of my life, and I find myself doing iRest even as I'm talking to people. I used to take Valium to feel okay. I'm so surprised that I can handle myself now without the Valium. I'm still falling asleep during my practice—and don't know how or why this practice works. But all I can say is, "I want more iRest."

iRest Nap

Imagine something that you could easily take that would increase your alertness and creativity; reduce your stress; improve your perception, stamina, and motor skills; enhance your sex life; help you make better decisions; keep you looking younger; help you lose weight; reduce the risk of having a heart attack; elevate your mood; strengthen your memory; and help heal your PTSD. Surprisingly, this miracle drug is a daily nap (Mednick and Erhman 2006). An iRest nap includes all of the benefits above, as well as all the ones we discuss throughout this book. So, as Sara Mednick says in the title of her book on napping, *Take a nap and change your life.*

Practice 26: 12-Minute Healing Nap

The following practice invites you to enter into a relaxed state of mind and body. This healing nap provides all the benefits listed in the previous paragraph. It's one of the best things you can do each day to help heal your PTSD.

Intention

Begin by affirming that you're entering into a short, restful nap.... As you affirm this, welcome into your body and mind the felt-sense of your inner resource of ease and well-being....

With your eyes gently open or closed...welcome the environment and sounds around you...the sensation of air as it touches your skin...the sensations of your body touching the surface that's supporting you...your body breathing...the various sensations that are calling your attention in your body....

Bodysensing

Welcome the sensations of your jaw...mouth...ears...cheeks...nose...eyes.... Welcome the physical sensations that make up your eyes.... Allow the sensations of your physical eyes to gently flow and mingle with the sensations of your entire face, head, and neck.... Follow this flow of sensation down through your neck...down into your shoulders and arms...down into your chest and belly...down into your pelvis, legs, and feet.... Welcome your entire body as a field of radiant sensation....

Now bring attention to the felt-sense of your torso and heart area.... Welcome the feeling of joy in your heart.... Rather than looking with your physical eyes, feel as if you're looking out with the "eyes of your heart."... Sense your entire body and the world around you with the eyes of your heart...front and back...left and right...your entire body....

Welcome sensations in your jaw...mouth...ears...nose...eyes...forehead...scalp...neck...shoulders...arms...hands...both arms and hands at the same time...the entire torso...front and back...releasing thinking...just sensing...your entire torso...both legs and feet at the same time...the entire body, inside and outside, as a field of sensation....

Enjoy, in a relaxed manner, the state you find yourself in...your body and mind deeply resting or sleeping, even as you find yourself present and aware.... Remain here as long as you wish...just being...at ease...just being...just being.

iRest for Sleep

The following practice is a wonderful way to fall asleep or get back to sleep. By working with this practice each time you fall asleep, you create a routine that conditions your body and mind to easily fall into deep, restful sleep.

Practice 27: iRest for Sleep

Begin by affirming that you're now entering into a deep, restful sleep.... As you affirm this to yourself, welcome into your body and mind the felt-sense of your inner resource of ease and well-being....

Allow your senses to open to the environment and sounds around you... the sensation of air touching your skin...the sensations of your body touching the surface that's supporting you.... Welcome your body breathing...the various physical sensations that are present...letting go into the feeling of being...being at ease throughout your entire body and mind....

Breathsensing

Bring your attention to the sensation of your body breathing...just noting... without getting involved...like you're on a raft floating gently on a stream of sensation...noting your body breathing...the coming and going of each inhalation and exhalation...your belly releasing with each exhalation...feeling yourself relaxing and letting go with each exhalation...with each exhalation, noting the belly softening...releasing...relaxing...letting go into the felt-sense of ease and well-being....

Welcome and nourish the sensation of your inner resource of well-being, peace, and ease, as you continue noting your body breathing.... With each breath, welcome the feeling of well-being into every cell of your body....

Bodysensing

With each exhalation, welcome sensation throughout your body while you feel yourself letting go into deep, restful sleep.... Welcome the sensations of your jaw...mouth...tongue...roof of the mouth...bottom of the mouth... side walls.... Give up thinking and welcome sensation in the entire jaw and mouth....

Exhale...sensing your left ear...right ear...the sensation of both ears at the same time....

Exhale...sensing your cheeks...nose...the flow of sensation inside both nostrils....

Exhale...sensing your left eye...right eye...the sensation of both eyes at the same time.... Give up thinking...simply feel your way....

Exhale...sensing your forehead...cool and relaxed...scalp...back of the head...neck...at rest and at ease....

Sense your left shoulder...left upper arm...elbow...forearm...wrist... hand...fingers...your entire left arm...heavy...relaxed...at ease....

Sense your right shoulder...right upper arm...elbow...forearm...wrist... hand...fingers...your entire right arm...heavy...relaxed...at ease....

Give up thinking.... Welcome both arms and hands at the same time....

Bring attention into the upper chest...upper back...midback...midchest... belly...lower back...the entire torso, front and back, as sensation.... Let go of thinking.... Sense and feel your way...with each exhalation, your entire torso heavy and relaxed...warm and at ease....

Sense your pelvis...left hip...left thigh...knee...lower leg...ankle, foot, and toes...the entire left leg heavy, relaxed, and at ease...your entire body heavy, relaxed, and at ease....

Sense your right hip...right thigh...right knee...lower leg...ankle, foot, and toes...the entire right leg heavy, relaxed, and at ease...your entire body relaxed, heavy...at ease....

Sense both legs at the same time...both legs heavy...relaxed...at ease....

Sense the entire front of the body...back of the body...left side of the body...right side of the body...sensation inside the body...sensation on the surface of the body...with each exhalation, your entire body relaxed, heavy... at ease....

Sense your breathing and heartbeat, slow...steady...regular...your entire body relaxed...heavy...at ease....

Well-Being

Sense well-being...peace...relaxation spreading throughout your entire body...with every exhalation, sensations of warmth, ease, heaviness, and well-being radiating throughout your entire body...head...arms and hands... torso...legs and feet...well-being, peace, and deep relaxation throughout your entire body....

Everywhere

Allow your attention to let go into all directions at once...inside...outside... everywhere at once.... Welcome the feeling of simply being...relaxed...at

ease...simply being...enjoying restful relaxation and the ease of being...
your body and mind deeply resting...just being...at ease...just being...just
being....

Use this practice regularly at night to help you enter into deep and
restful sleep. By practicing regularly, you train your body to fall asleep
easily and quickly. If you find yourself waking up in the middle of the
night, use this practice to support your body and mind to fall back again
into restful sleep. If, as you're falling asleep, you experience a particular
emotion or thought getting in your way of going to sleep, take time to work
with the iRest tools Affirming Your Inner Resource, Welcoming Opposites
of Feeling and Emotion, and Welcoming Opposites of Thought. Each tool
of iRest helps your body and mind establish a routine that you can depend
on to help you fall asleep at night, no matter your circumstance or
situation.

Inviting Gratitude into Your Life

It's important for your healing, health, and well-being to experience
regular and random moments of joy throughout your day. An effective way
to enhance your ability to experience joy is to spend time taking *gratitude
moments*. Gratitude moments take place when you welcome the felt-sense
of gratitude and give thanks for things in your life. You do this by taking a
few minutes four to six times each day, especially before going to sleep, to
recall what you're thankful for. Or take time to write letters to people
you're grateful to. It's not necessary for you to actually send the letters you
write. Just the act of writing and expressing your gratitude is enough.
Research shows that people who regularly take time during their day for
gratitude are much happier and less depressed months later than those
who do not engage in gratitude practices (Emmons and McCullough 2003;
Grant and Gino 2010; Lambert and Fincham 2011; Sansone and Sansone
2010; Seligman et al. 2005).

Take time each day, before taking an iRest nap, or before going to
sleep at night, to reflect on and even write down in your journal one to
three things that you're grateful for and why. Notice where and how you
experience gratitude (in your heart, belly, throat, etc.). As you experience

gratitude in your body, slowly let go of what you're grateful for and simply rest in the feeling of gratitude. Stay with this feeling of gratitude as you go about your day, take a nap, or fall asleep at night. It's also helpful to welcome the feeling of gratitude as you're waking up in the morning, before heading into your day.

Practice 28: Welcoming Gratitude

Now you will welcome the feeling of gratitude in your body. You can do this same practice with other qualities such as love, kindness, compassion, peace, joy, or any other positive emotion that comes to mind.

Allow your senses to open to the environment and sounds around you... the sensation where the air touches your skin...the sensation where your body touches the surface that's supporting you.... Welcome your body breathing...' the various physical sensations that are present...letting go into the feeling of being...being at ease throughout your entire body and mind....

Welcoming Gratitude

Notice feelings of gratitude that are present in your mind and body...perhaps gratitude for a friend or animal in your life; or gratitude for where you live; or gratitude for something someone has done for you; or gratitude for having food, a home, and clothing; or gratitude for no reason at all...just grati-tude.... Welcome in the feeling of gratitude and any accompanying feelings like joy, ease, or contentment so that gratitude spreads throughout your entire body as a physical reality.... As you're welcoming gratitude, allow your heart to grow warm with an inner smile that spreads up into your lips, eyes, and face...feeling gratitude with your entire body.... Allow the feeling of gratitude to expand so that you feel it radiating into the space all around you....

Notice opposite feelings that may arise, such as disappointment...loss... or feelings of sadness or unhappiness.... If opposites arise, welcome them, then, in turn, welcome in the feeling of gratitude...allowing both to be here at the same time, as well as your inner resource of well-being and ease of being.... Allow the feeling of gratitude to fill in any feelings of emptiness... allowing gratitude to touch all the parts of you that feel or have felt unhappy at one time.... As it feels right, let go of any negative opposites and stay with the feeling of gratitude.... Allow yourself to feel gratitude for no reason at all...just the feeling of gratitude....

Completion

As you come to feel complete with this exercise and are ready to return to your day and activities, affirm your intention to take the feeling of gratitude with you into your life.... Affirm that all day long you welcome gratitude.... Let gratitude accompany you in every activity and interaction.... As you're ready, open and close your eyes several times while feeling gratitude throughout your body and mind.... Then, go about your activities knowing that gratitude is always there, remembering you all day, every day, wherever you are, whatever you're doing, whomever you're with.

Moving Forward

You don't have to change your circumstance to experience joy. iRest teaches you to recognize and feel joy in the midst of its opposites. Whether you're experiencing happiness or sorrow, peace or conflict, comfort or pain, being and joy are always present. Being and joy fill and surround every experience.

In this chapter, I discussed how iRest reveals two types of joy: (1) joy that comes with an experience, and (2) joy that exists independent of whatever else is present. Take time throughout each and every day to experience being and joy. Through this daily practice, you can experience being and joy as always present in the midst of both the stressful and easeful events of your life. Feeling being and joy allows you to stay connected to yourself and the world around you. The good news is that you don't have to wait for PTSD to be healed to feel joy and being. But taking time to welcome joy and being in your body and mind does help heal your PTSD.

Chapter 10

Being Awareness

I found it hard to come back and live a normal life after being in combat. iRest helped calm my soul. It gave me a break from my injuries and memories of brothers I'd lost. To just close my eyes, take a break from life, breathe in relaxation, and be in peace helped me remember who I am. At first I didn't get it. But the more I practiced, the more I experienced my life changing for the better. I truly believe that iRest saved my life. It gave me the hope and strength I needed to reconnect to myself and to the world again.

—Gulf War veteran

iRest tools #1 through #8 focus on individual messengers of sensations, emotions, and thoughts that arise *in* your awareness. In this chapter you'll learn how iRest tool #9, Being Awareness, invites you to shift your focus to *awareness* itself. With this tool, you'll learn to shift your attention from individual details to the whole picture.

Allow me to explain with this metaphor: During your practice of iRest tools #1 through #8, you've been invited to focus on the individual clouds (emotions, thoughts, etc.) that are present in the sky (awareness). iRest tool #9 invites you to experience and welcome the sky itself—yourself as awareness. Your ability to welcome and experience yourself as awareness is the ultimate tool to help you attain optimal healing and health. So, along with welcoming your heartfelt mission, intentions, inner resource, sensations, emotions, thoughts, and joy, in this chapter you learn to fully welcome yourself as the field of awareness in which all these other sensations and movements arise.

iRest Tool #9: Being Awareness

Let's stay with the example of clouds and sky. Imagine yourself as the sky. As the sky, you are aware of the trees, the smells in the air, and the sound of the birds. In this way, you're aware of the things around you that are *in* the spaciousness of the sky.

Let's use the room in which you're reading this book as another example. You're aware of this book, the words on this page, and the various objects around you. This book, these words, and all of the objects around you are *in* your awareness. You're also aware of your thoughts, sensations, and emotions. Each of these is also *in* your awareness. Everything you experience is *in* your awareness. Many of us have never considered this, but it's true.

Let's get started! Here's a practice that's designed to give you the experience of *being* awareness. However you choose to go through this practice, take time to pause and fully experience each step before moving on.

Practice 29: Being Awareness 1

Adjust your body so that you feel completely supported by the surface on which you're resting.... Scan your body and release any unnecessary tension...senses open to your environment and the sounds around you....

With your eyes open, bring your attention to a particular object that's in the space around you.... Focus your attention only on this one object....

Note its size...color...shape...and form....

Note particular thoughts or feelings you have about this object....

Now, soften your eyes.... Allow your attention to defocus.... Without focusing on any particular object, take in all of the objects around you....

Instead of looking with your eyes, feel with your entire body as you take in all of the objects around you without focusing on any particular object....

Experience the space around you...in front...behind...to your left... right...inside...outside.... Experience yourself simply being...not focusing on any particular external object...just being...attention relaxed...eyes soft... eyes open or closed...just being.... ·

Note that you're aware of the felt-sense of being.... You can feel yourself being.... You're aware of the objects around you and the sensations within your body and mind.... Note how you're aware of everything.... Note that everything you're experiencing is in your awareness.... Everything is in your awareness....

Gently feel into awareness.... What does awareness feel like?... Let your eyes stay soft and your thinking mind stay relaxed and at ease.... Sense how everything is arising within your awareness...objects...the sense of space...being...how you're aware of everything you're experiencing...and how you're aware of awareness.... Sense awareness...not by looking at awareness but by feeling, sensing, and being awareness...feeling...sensing...being awareness....

Note how your attention becomes involved with thinking or with an object or sensation that's arising in your field of awareness.... Welcome thinking or whatever else may arise in your awareness.... Keep returning to the felt-sense of being awareness....

Go back and forth between noting thoughts or other sensations or objects that you're aware of...and awareness itself.... Sense and feel what it's like to be the field of awareness in which all these movements of your body, mind, and senses are arising and passing away....

Take your time.... Note an object that's in your awareness...then, feel into being awareness....

When you feel ready, open and close your eyes several times while continuing to feel yourself being awareness.... Then, take a few minutes to record in your journal words that best describe what it's like being awareness.

The Importance of Being Awareness

Why is being awareness so important? By learning to shift your attention from the experience you're having to being awareness, you can instantly gain a wider view of everything you're experiencing. By getting perspective on what you're experiencing, you're able to attain understanding and recognize actions you need to take that you might otherwise miss when you don't have perspective.

You've probably heard the expression "Keep things in perspective." This expression speaks to your ability to see the sky, not just the clouds. You can lose sight of the sky when you become too focused on a particular sensation, emotion, thought, or symptom of PTSD. By shifting your attention from the object (sensation, emotion, thought, or symptom) that's *in* your awareness to *being* awareness, you have at your fingertips a powerful tool that you can use to instantly gain a broader view of whatever you're experiencing. When you learn to *be* awareness, you learn how not to get caught up in your experience. When you don't get caught up in your experience, you're able to maintain distance from and gain perspective *on* your experience. Distance from your experience allows you to see actions you need to take to help you move through everything you experience in life, including your symptoms of PTSD. As a way to help deepen your understanding of why it's important to learn how to be awareness, let me share Jonathan's story with you.

> *Since returning from his tour of duty two years ago, Jonathan's been in a major depression. When I ask him to describe what he's experiencing, he says he feels sad and hopeless, paralyzed by guilt and self-judgment, and a lack of energy and motivation. As Jonathan describes how he feels, I ask him to take note of each feeling he's describing. Then, I invite him to note that he's aware of each feeling as he describes it to me. I point out to him that he can't describe what he's feeling unless he's aware of it. His awareness is what allows Jonathan to describe what he's feeling. This is the beginning of Jonathan's understanding that each and every thing he's experiencing is arising in his awareness.*
>
> *Building on this understanding, I invite Jonathan to experiment with shifting his attention from a specific experience to awareness itself. First, I guide him to note an emotion he's aware of. Jonathan notes his sadness. Then, I invite him to note awareness itself. We continue in this way, slowly going through Jonathan's list of emotions, thoughts, et cetera, item by item. For each, I ask Jonathan to sense the particular emotion or thought he's having, to note that he's aware of it, then to describe his felt-sense of awareness.*
>
> *From there, I invite Jonathan to shift his attention from resting in awareness to resting as awareness. To help him understand the difference between resting in awareness and resting as awareness, I explain that resting as awareness is like*

settling into a bathtub of warm water. At first he feels himself in the water, then he merges with and becomes the water.

As Jonathan shifts his attention to resting as awareness, I ask him to describe what's happening in his body and mind. He reports that he feels a shift within himself from being in his depression to his depression being in his awareness. He reports feeling more relaxed and at ease, and feeling a lessening of his depression as a result of this shift within himself.

As Jonathan and I continue working together, he spends less time lost in the feeling of his depression. He develops his ability to rest as awareness for longer periods of time. As he takes time being awareness, he uncovers an underlying feeling of joy that he hadn't known before.

Jonathan reports that the feeling of freedom he experiences in my office gives him a sense of hope that he can find his way through his depression. Through his growing ability to rest as awareness, Jonathan's able to take breaks from and gain perspective on his depression. As he continues practicing iRest, Jonathan learns to welcome the messengers that lie hidden within his depression. Slowly but surely, this process supports Jonathan to take the actions that allow him to break free of his depression.

Awareness and Well-Being

The goal of each tool of iRest is to teach you to experience a deep and stable sense of well-being within yourself. During your early experiences with iRest, well-being can feel like an unsteady and short-lived experience that comes and goes. As you grow in your ability to welcome your emotions and thoughts, you also grow in your ability to rest as being. Resting as being develops your capacity to experience well-being as a more steady and stable state. In turn, it becomes the step you use to experience yourself as awareness. Resting as awareness opens you to experiencing an indestructible sense of well-being and a non-separate wholeness with all of life.

Whether you're aware of awareness or not, awareness is present in every moment. Awareness always is. It cannot be disturbed, no matter your circumstance or situation. Awareness is the ultimate ground from which your inner resource of true safety, security, well-being, and joy emerges. Resting as awareness reveals a quality of well-being that's steady, stable, and unchanging. Awareness *is* your ultimate inner resource.

Being Versus Awareness

At this point, you may be wondering how *being* is different from *awareness*. Good question! Together, let's explore how awareness is different from the feeling that comes when you defocus your attention and rest as being.

Like every experience you have, the sense of defocusing and of being are experiences that arise *within* your awareness. Awareness is unlike any other experience you have. Awareness isn't an object. You can't look at awareness in the same way you look at a thought, emotion, sensation, your symptoms of PTSD, the feeling of being, or other objects in the world around you. Awareness isn't an object arising in something. Awareness contains everything, including itself! Without awareness you wouldn't know any "thing." Every "thing," every object, comes and goes in awareness. Every sensation, emotion, and thought comes and goes *in* awareness. Your feeling focused or defocused comes and goes *in* awareness. And your felt-sense of being, and even self-awareness, comes and goes *in* awareness. Every single experience you have comes and goes in awareness. However, awareness doesn't come and go. It's not an object. Because awareness isn't an object, you can't look at awareness as you would an object. Awareness just is. To know awareness, you need to be awareness!

The practice of iRest reveals that awareness is forever unchanging and always present. Awareness is the sky in which every cloud of your experience appears and disappears.

Practice 30: Qualities of Awareness

In order to get a better handle on why awareness is such a valuable tool, let's explore some of the important qualities of awareness.

Adjust your body so that you feel completely supported by the surface on which you're resting...senses open to your environment and the sounds around you.... Scan your body and release any unnecessary tension.... Allow your body to settle...your mind to relax and be at ease.... Now, reflect on the following words and feel the truth of each statement. Feel the truth with your feeling heart, not your thinking brain.

I'm aware of my body, mind, and senses. These are movements arising in awareness.

I'm aware of the world around me. The world is a movement arising in awareness.

I'm aware of the movement of attention. Attention is a movement in awareness.

I'm aware of being self-aware. Self-awareness is a movement in awareness.

I know myself and the world around me because awareness is.

Everything arises within, moves within, and disappears within awareness.

Everything is in awareness. Awareness contains everything.

Remove all objects and awareness still is.

Awareness is everywhere.

Awareness is here before, during, and after whatever arises in awareness.

Awareness surrounds, touches, and fills everything.

Awareness is empty. Because it's empty, awareness is able to contain everything.

Awareness is formless and indescribable, yet undeniable.

All objects are free to come and go in awareness.

Awareness doesn't refuse, reject, attach, or hold on to anything.

Awareness "welcomes" everything.

Awareness is welcoming.

I am awareness.

Now, let all of these statements fall into the background.... Let all objects (sensations, emotions, thoughts, etc.) that are in awareness, including the feeling of being, fall into the background.... With all of these objects in the background, let awareness come into the foreground.... Be aware of awareness.... Notice that you're aware of awareness.... Now feel yourself relaxing into being awareness...resting as awareness.... Feel the effect that resting as awareness has on your body and mind. Take your time....

Keep feeling yourself as awareness and look around at objects in your immediate environment.... Note each object that your eyes land on and feel yourself being awareness at the same time.... What's this like to realize yourself as awareness, even as you gaze upon different objects?...

Try this practice with a physical sensation.... Experience a particular sensation—for example, comfort or discomfort—and feel yourself as awareness at the same time.... Try the same practice with an emotion and a thought.... What's it like to feel yourself as awareness as you go about your day?...

When you're ready, open and close your eyes several times while continuing to feel yourself being awareness.... With your eyes open, notice objects in the environment around you, all the while being awareness.... If it feels comfortable, get up and walk around your environment, all the while staying with the felt-sense of being awareness.... Then, go about your day while noticing how the felt-sense of being awareness is always here as a background presence....

Take time to reflect on each experiment you make. Then, take time to record your reflections in your journal.

Your Core Identity Is Awareness

You've learned to think of yourself as a separate individual. You've learned to believe that you're separate, unique, and distinct; that there's no one else exactly like you. While this is true, it's only half of the story. The opposite is also true. There's something about you that's not separate, distinct, or unique. Your core identity—what you are beyond all the sensations, emotions, and thoughts of your body and mind, and what you share in common with all others—is awareness. Your core identity, like everyone around you, is awareness—the awareness in which all your sensations, emotions, and thoughts, and all your symptoms of PTSD, arise.

When you believe only half the story—that you are only your body and mind—you identify with the sensations of your body and the movements of your mind. Rather than saying, *Painful sensation is present,* you say, *I have a headache.* Rather than saying, *Anger is present,* you say, *I'm angry.* Rather than saying, *The thought is present that something's wrong,* you say, *Something's wrong with me.* Holding the belief that you're only your sensations, emotions, or thoughts causes you to be overly identified with and wrapped up in your sensations, emotions, and thoughts.

Resting as awareness allows you to recognize that you're something much more than any of the sensations, emotions, or thoughts you have, including your symptoms of PTSD. Because all your symptoms of PTSD arise in awareness, resting as awareness allows you to see that you're something greater than any of your symptoms of PTSD. This knowledge empowers you to come to the deepest healing of your PTSD.

Your Sense of Self

Everything that you're aware of comes and goes in your awareness. Each of these objects that comes and goes is "claimed" by the thought *I*, which we'll call the *I-thought*. Your I-thought attaches to and fuses with whatever you're experiencing. You say, "I'm hungry," "I have a headache," "I'm tired," "I'm anxious," or "I'm sad." However, these statements don't describe your actual experience. It's more accurate to describe your experience as "Hunger is present," "Sensation of pain is present," "The feeling of fatigue is present," and "Emotions of anxiety or sadness are present." You're used to fusing with the experiences that come and go in your life. But have you ever asked about the nature of this I-thought that attaches to your experiences? Who or what is this "I" that keeps attaching to every sensation, thought, and emotion?

iRest tool #9, Being Awareness, invites you to explore the nature of this I-thought, which you identify with and take yourself to be. The practice of iRest is designed to help you understand:

- The difference between the objects that are coming and going in your awareness

- The I-thought that fuses with these comings and goings

- Awareness, in which everything, including the I-thought, is coming and going

The natural tendency of your mind is to fuse with the thought *I*. Your mind then believes that you're a separate self (Baumann and Taft 2011; Eagleman 2011; Metzinger 2009). The practice of iRest invites you to understand that the I-thought is just another thought or object that's arising *in* awareness. This understanding breaks your mind's fusion with the I-thought. As you break your fusion with the I-thought, your belief that you're only a separate and distinct self collapses (Baumann and Taft

2011; Eagleman 2011; Metzinger 2009). The following practice invites you to experience this for yourself.

Practice 31: Entering the Stream of Awareness

Adjust your body so that you feel completely supported by the surface on which you're resting...senses wide open to your environment and the sounds around you.... Scan your body and release any unnecessary tension.... Welcome your inner resource and the feelings of ease and well-being throughout your entire body and mind....

Become aware of a sensation, emotion, or thought that's present in your body or mind.... Notice how the I-thought appears and accompanies whatever you're aware of.... For example, "I'm aware of this sensation," or "I'm aware of this emotion," or "I'm aware of this thought."

Now, turn your attention to being aware of this I-thought.... As you do this, repeat silently to yourself, I...I...I.... Experience your felt-sense of this I-thought.... As you repeat I, notice how a new I-thought appears to witness the I-thought that's being silently repeated.... Notice this "new" I-thought, and observe how a new I-thought appears to witness it, too.... As you continue, notice how all these movements of "I" are appearing in your awareness....

Begin to shift your attention away from being fused with the I-thought to your felt-sense of being awareness.... Shift your attention from being a distinct "I" (focusing network) to simply being awareness (defocusing network).... Experience yourself as the expansive and spacious openness of awareness....

Feel yourself being awareness and note that there's still a subtle I-thought that's present.... Sense how this I-thought is arising in the vast field of awareness, which has no I-thought attached to it....

Sense how awareness surrounds and fills everything that's arising, including the feeling of you being a distinct "I."... Let go of what's arising in awareness, what's coming and going in awareness, and feel yourself dissolving into simply being awareness...awareness that exists before your mind identifies with the thought I and separates what is indivisible into a separate self, other, and world....

Take time being awareness.... Notice how your mind drifts away at times into a thought, emotion, or sensation.... Notice how the I-thought automatically arises and fuses with whatever is present.... When you notice that this is happening, you don't need to change anything.... Simply notice that all this is arising in awareness.... Then, welcome your felt-sense of being awareness.... Notice how awareness is always present, even when your mind is involved with something other than being awareness....

When you're ready, open and close your eyes several times while continuing to feel yourself being awareness.... With your eyes open, notice objects in the environment around you, all the while being awareness.... If it feels comfortable, get up and walk around your environment, all the while staying with the felt-sense of being awareness.... Then, go about your day while noticing how the felt-sense of being awareness is always there as a background presence.

Infinite Regression

The process of "I" noticing "I" noticing "I" is called an *infinite regression*. It's similar to what happens when you stand between two mirrors, one in front and one behind you. The mirrors create the illusion that your image goes on forever.

Your sense of being a separate self or "I" is dependent on your thinking mind. Your thinking mind, like two mirrors facing one another, keeps in place the belief of being a separate "I." When you recognize that your every thought, including your I-thought, is simply an object arising in your awareness, your identification with your belief in being a separate self or "I" is set free to be there as just a thought. It's just a thought arising *in* awareness. As your attention moves from being fused with the I-thought, you can rest more and more as awareness. Resting as awareness dissolves your felt-sense of being separate. As this happens, you experience yourself as being empty yet full, without form yet undeniable, separate yet connected. You experience your basic foundation of interconnected wholeness that you share with all others and the world around you. You also discover that your non-separate and interconnected wholeness is incapable of being harmed by any symptom of PTSD. This is where you find your ultimate inner resource of health, wholeness, and unchanging well-being. This unchanging well-being is always unharmed by anything you experience, ever.

Who, What, Why, When, and Where Am I?

Remember English class? In helping you write papers, your teacher might have taught you to ask, Who? What? Why? When? Where? Like your English teacher, iRest invites you to ask these same questions. However, iRest invites you to ask these questions as a means to exploring and challenging your belief that you are a separate "I" by asking, *Who am I? What am I? Why am I? When am I? Where am I?*

Generally speaking, exploring the answers to these questions is important in four ways:

1. It dissolves your identification with the I-thought.

2. It dissolves your belief in being a separate self.

3. It leads to your experiencing yourself as an interconnected part of the whole.

4. It lays the groundwork for healing your symptoms of PTSD.

More specific to healing your symptoms of PTSD, exploring the answers to these questions dissolves anxiety, fear, and suffering that prevents final resolution of your PTSD (Baumann and Taft 2011; Metzinger 2009).

Who or what is this "I" that's experiencing all of these changing movements of body, mind, senses, and world? Who or what is aware of these sensations of the body and flows of energy? Who or what is aware of these emotions, thoughts, and images? Who or what is this "I" that is aware? Asking these questions and following them to answers reveals that everything is a non-separate part, or expression, of awareness. There is no separate self or "I." Your sense of self or "I" is just another thought arising in awareness. Everything arises in, and is a non-separate expression of, awareness. Ultimately, there is only awareness.

When all sense of self and "I" dissolve completely there is only awareness. Awareness is who you are. Awareness is what you are. Awareness is why you are. Awareness is when you are. Awareness is where you are. You are the spacious, timeless, perfect, complete, and unchanging health and wholeness of awareness.

When you are truly resting *as* awareness, there is no separate "I" who is experiencing something. When you truly recognize and rest as aware-ness, there's only awareness without anyone who is aware. This is called *cessation*. It's similar to when you're in deep sleep, without experiencing any thoughts regarding the world or yourself.

The deepest experience of iRest brings you to moments of cessation. When your sense of being an individual, separate self returns from moments of cessation, you feel different from when you've simply fallen into deep sleep. You return from these moments sensing the "perfume" of where you just were. This is the perfume of pure awareness. You return from moments of pure awareness with a deep sense of the wholeness that you truly are—your true identity. Knowing pure awareness as your true identity allows you to dive more deeply into feeling your core identity as deep peace, contentment, and well-being that can never be disturbed, no matter what. This knowledge allows you to welcome and fully heal your PTSD.

Practice 32: Being Awareness 2

The first phase of the following practice involves the process of de-fusing or dis-identifying from all that you believe you are, whether body, senses, or mind. This first phase consists of three parts, which deal with the physical, emotional, and mental aspects of your body and mind. De-fusion or dis-identification from the I-thought leads to the second phase of this exercise, which is the realization of your essential identity as awareness.

De-fusion leads to the understanding and insight that who you actually are is far more than your belief and feeling of being a separate self or "I." Freeing yourself from the belief that you're separate leads to experiencing unchanging well-being, health, and wholeness.

This practice allows your mind to defocus. As your mind defocuses, you're able to recognize your sense of being. Resting as being reveals aware-ness. Resting as awareness brings freedom from identification with the ever-changing phenomena of your body and mind. Freedom from these changing phenomena gives rise to freedom from pain, anxiety, fear, and suffering. Freedom from these states of mind and body, along with the recognition of your underlying, unchanging health and well-being, paves the way for healing your PTSD.

Resting as awareness creates space within you from which it's easier to see and welcome actions you need to take to heal your PTSD. Resting as awareness allows you to recognize and welcome your natural feelings of self-power. It enhances your ability to respond, which enables you to move beyond your sense of powerlessness. Resting as awareness allows you to stay grounded and able to respond to others and the world around you, no matter your circumstance or situation.

Rather than think your way through the following practice, you're invited to feel your way through it. To understand the difference between feeling and thinking, imagine entering a completely dark room that's filled with furniture. In order to find your way to the other side of the room, you need to suspend thinking and feel your way around the furniture. Throughout the following practice, reflect on and experience the effect of each statement slowly and thoughtfully with your feeling body and heart, rather than with your thinking mind.

Settling In

Adjust your body so that you feel completely supported by the surface on which you're resting.... Open your senses and welcome the environment and sounds around you.... Scan your body and release any unnecessary tension.... Welcome your inner resource and the feeling of ease or well-being throughout your entire body and mind....

Now that your body is at rest, silently say the following statements to yourself. Go slowly. Take time with each statement. Feel how each statement impacts your body, breath, and mind. Move on to the next statement only when you feel complete with the statement you're on.

Body

I have a body, but I am not just my body. I am the one who is aware of my body.

My body finds itself in different conditions of health and sickness. I value my body as a precious instrument of experience and action. I treat my body well and seek to keep it in good health.

I have a body, but I am not just my body. I am the one who is aware of my body.... Take time to register and feel this statement as your actual experience. I have a body, but I am not just my body. I am the one who is aware of my body.

When you're ready, move on to the next part of this practice.

Emotions

I have emotions, but I am not just my emotions. I am the one who is aware of my emotions.

My emotions are varied, changing, and sometimes contradictory. They can change from calm to anger, from joy to sorrow, and yet my essence as awareness does not change. Though a wave of anger or sadness may temporarily submerge me, I know that it will pass in time. Therefore, I am not just my emotions.

Since I can be aware of and notice my emotions, it is clear that I am not just my emotions.

I have emotions, but I am not just my emotions. I am the one who is aware of my emotions.... Take time to register and feel this statement as your actual experience.... I have emotions, but I am not just my emotions. I am the one who is aware of my emotions.

When you're ready, move on to the next part of this practice.

Thoughts

I have thoughts, but I am not just my thoughts. I am the one who is aware of my thoughts.

My thoughts are a valuable tool of discovery and expression, but they are not the essence of who and what I truly am. My thoughts are constantly changing as my mind embraces new ideas, knowledge, and experience.

I have thoughts, but I am not just my thoughts. I am the one who is aware of my thoughts.... Take time to register and feel this statement as your actual experience.... *I have thoughts, but I am not just my thoughts. I am the one who is aware of my thoughts.* When you're ready, move on to the next part of this practice.

Unchanging Awareness

Now, slowly affirm and feel each of the following statements.

I have a body, but I am not just my body. I am the one who is aware of my body.

I have emotions, but I am not just my emotions. I am the one who is aware of my emotions.

I have thoughts, but I am not just my thoughts. I am the one who is aware of my thoughts.

I am unchanging awareness, in which the ever-changing flow of my life arises.... Take time to register and feel this statement as your actual experience.... *I am unchanging awareness, in which the ever-changing flow of my life arises.*

When you're ready, move on to the next part of this practice.

I recognize and affirm that my essential nature is unchanging awareness. I recognize myself as awareness in the midst of my everyday life. I am unchanging awareness, in which the ever-changing flow of my life arises. Awareness is the ultimate source and inner resource that gives rise to meaning, purpose, and direction in my life.

Notice the changing movements of your body and mind.... Notice the unchanging nature of awareness. Take time now to rest as unchanging awareness....

When you're ready to return to your daily life, open and close your eyes several times while noticing objects in the environment around you, all the while resting as awareness.... As you begin to move, walk around your environment, all the while staying with the felt-sense of being awareness. Then, go about your day while noticing how the felt-sense of being unchanging awareness is always present as a background presence.

The previous exercise is most effective when you practice it daily, preferably during the first hours of your day. Whenever possible, do this practice as you're waking up. Consider the practice as a symbolic *second awakening*. It's of great value to repeat this practice throughout your day. To help make it easy and quick for you to do this, use the shorthand statement *I am unchanging awareness, in which the ever-changing flow of my life arises*. Or simply say to yourself, *Unchanging awareness.*

Each time you say and experience this statement, allow it to return you to your essential nature as unchanging awareness.

The longer version of Practice 32 can be modified to fit whatever sensation, emotion, or thought you may be currently experiencing. For instance, you could address *desires* you have or *roles* you play:

- **Desire:** *I have desires, but I am not just my desires. I am the one who is aware of my desires. My desires are constantly changing and sometimes contradictory. I have desires, but I am not just my desires. I am unchanging awareness, in which the ever-changing flow of my desires arises.*

- **Roles**: *I play many roles in life. I must play these roles, and I willingly play them as well as possible, be it the role of child, parent, friend, peer, lover, or spouse. I am aware that I am playing these roles. Therefore I am not just the roles I am playing. I am unchanging awareness, in which the ever-changing flow of my life arises.*

Additional Practices on Being Awareness

The following exercises—Who Am I? and I Am—are variations on the theme of welcoming and experiencing yourself as awareness.

Practice 33: Who Am I?

Adjust your body so that you feel completely supported by the surface on which you're resting.... Open your senses and welcome the environment and sounds around you.... Scan your body and release any unnecessary tension.... Welcome your inner resource and the feelings of ease and well-being throughout your entire body and mind....

Body

Take a few minutes to feel and sense your body.... Where is it comfortable?... Where is it uncomfortable?... Be aware of the various sensations that are present in your face...head...neck...shoulders...arms...hands...front of the torso...back of the torso...abdomen...pelvis...legs...feet.... Sense your heartbeat...your body breathing.... Now, gently ask yourself, *Who is aware?... What is aware?...*

Feelings and Emotions

Now, sense your state of feelings and emotions.... Without going into thinking, sense the feelings and emotions that are present.... Open yourself to obvious and subtle feelings and emotions....

If it's helpful, recall feelings and emotions that you experienced earlier today or during your week.... Now, gently ask yourself, *Who is aware of these feelings and emotions?... What is aware of these feelings and emotions?...*

Thoughts

Notice what you're thinking and how your thoughts follow one another.... When you realize you've been distracted by a thought, notice where you went and what brought you back.... Then, gently ask, *Who is aware of these thoughts?... What is aware of these thoughts?...*

Senses

Turn your attention to the environment around you.... Notice the temperature of the air...smells...sounds...the feeling of the surface that's supporting your body.... Allow your attention to expand out beyond your immediate environment.... Be aware of what is present in the surrounding neighborhood and beyond...in the countryside and beyond...in the world and beyond.... Sense the sun, moon, and stars.... Sense the entire universe.... Gently ask, *Who is aware of this body, the space around this body, the universe?... What is aware of this body, the space around this body, the universe?...*

Give time to experience yourself as being awareness.... Then, record your reflections in your journal.

The previous awareness practices, as well as the one that follows, are adapted from exercises that have been time-tested over thousands of years. Be patient with each, as any one practice may at first feel intellectual. But with time, each will deeply affect you and become your ally, helping you heal your PTSD.

Practice 34: I Am

Adjust your body so that you feel completely supported by the surface on which you're resting.... Open your senses and welcome the environment and sounds around you.... Scan your body and release any unnecessary tension.... Welcome your inner resource and the feeling of ease or well-being throughout your entire body and mind....

Sensing I Am

Sense an object that's in your awareness.
Now ask the question, *Who or what is aware of this object?*
The answer quite simply is: *I am.*
Experience the felt-sense of "I am" in your body...in your heart.
Now let the word "am" drop away.
Feel only the sense of "I" in your heart.
Now drop the word "I."
Just be, before the thought *I* arises.
Be with the stillness that remains.
Feel how you're aware of this stillness.
Allow the stillness to dissolve into awareness.
Be awareness before thoughts arise.
Allow the feeling of being awareness to expand from your heart into all directions.
Remain here being awareness.
When you're ready to go back into your daily life, open and close your eyes several times and begin to move your body while being awareness. As you move about in your daily life, experience how unchanging awareness is always present amidst your daily activities. Before moving on, take a few minutes to record your reflections in your journal.

You Are Love

iRest takes you beyond your usual identification with yourself as a separate self. The practice of iRest introduces you to your essential nature, which is awareness. Resting as awareness allows the feeling of love to emerge. As you awaken to your essential nature as awareness, unchanging love, compassion, self-kindness, and joy awaken as expressions of awareness.

When you don't know yourself as awareness, you can't recognize the underlying and unchanging love, compassion, kindness, and joy that are independent of your circumstances. Love is an essential quality of awareness. Awareness "loves" everything, because everything arises out of and melts back into awareness. Awareness has no judgment. Love, like awareness, has no judgment. Love calls you to welcome all the movements that arise within your body and mind without judgment. Love gives rise to the understanding that you're always doing the best you know how. Knowing this, you can relax and find the actions that help you heal your PTSD. True healing takes place not in self-judgment but in self-love, self-compassion, and self-kindness.

As your essential nature of awareness blossoms, love also blossoms. From awareness and love blossoms your ability to accept things as they are, as well as your ability to respond without defending, resisting, or refusing. Responding—rather than defending, resisting, or refusing—allows you to understand what you're experiencing, which leads you to the actions that enable you to heal your PTSD. Taking the actions you need to take to heal your PTSD restores harmony to your relationships and life. With harmony, you fully blossom in your life with purpose, meaning, and value.

Moving Forward

Knowing yourself and resting as unchanging awareness allows you to welcome your deepest heartfelt mission, intentions, and inner resource. Welcoming and experiencing your heartfelt mission, intentions, and inner resource supports your ability to utilize the tools of iRest that follow.

So, let us turn to the next chapter and discuss how experiencing your undivided wholeness may have escaped your attention. By doing this, you pave the way for recognizing and experiencing your wholeness for the rest of your life.

Chapter 11

Experiencing Your Wholeness

Through my practice of iRest, I now know this unchanging peace that's within me. I feel like a samurai warrior who finally knows the secret.

—Vietnam veteran

In chapters 4 through 9, you learned to welcome everything you experience. You learned how welcoming, rather than refusing, enables you to respond to what you're experiencing with actions that empower you to feel in harmony with yourself and the world. In chapter 10, you learned to shift your attention from being aware *of* what you're experiencing to welcoming yourself *as* awareness. As awareness, you gain perspective on everything you're experiencing. By *being* awareness, you're able to see the actions you need to take that you'd otherwise miss when you don't take up the perspective of being awareness. In this chapter, I show you how your ability to be awareness leads you to see and experience everything in the entire universe, including yourself, as a unique expression of the wholeness of life. In this chapter, you learn to experience yourself as a unique, but not separate, expression of the wholeness of life.

Unique and Not Separate

Your body, mind, emotions, and thoughts form a distinct pattern. You, like every person and thing, are a unique expression of life. However, this is only half the story. While your body is made up of separate parts, together they form a whole that is your body. Similarly, your skin defines the boundary of your body. It separates your body from the objects around you. However, look at your skin through an electron microscope and all sense of boundary dissolves. You can't tell where your skin ends and the world around you begins. Your body is actually not separate from the world around you. This is the same for every person and thing around you, and in the entire universe. From one perspective, we see parts. From another, we see only what is whole and not separate. The iRest program enables you to experience yourself as unique and non-separate. Through the practice, you learn to experience yourself as a unique individual who is, *at the same time*, interconnected and not separate from the wholeness of life. Experiencing yourself as whole and not separate is perhaps the most powerful healing practice within the iRest program. It's this that makes iRest such a vital program for healing your PTSD. You may not yet feel your wholeness, but you are—and always have been—whole, complete, unharmed, and healthy.

iRest Tool #10: Experiencing Your Wholeness

The iRest tool Experiencing Your Wholeness takes place in several phases. Let's learn about all six of them.

Phase 1

During the first phase, your attention is on *what* you're experiencing—be it sensation, feeling, emotion, or thought—as changing states of your body and mind. In this phase, you learn to be aware *of* and respond *to* these changing states. Being aware of these changing states as they arise allows you to acknowledge them. Acknowledging them keeps you from fusing with them and permits you to gain a broader view of your experiences. From this broad view, you're able to recognize how to respond with the right action to each changing state of your body and mind that you experience.

This first phase nourishes your ability to be aware *of*, stay connected *to*, but *not* fuse with what you're experiencing. This phase also supports you to develop your capacity for experiencing well-being and harmony within yourself and in all your interactions with others and the world.

Phase 2

During the second phase, your attention shifts from observing the changing states that are arising *in* your awareness to observing yourself *as* an observer who is aware *of* these changing states. Here, you learn to develop your knowledge of yourself as an observer who is observing. As you become aware of yourself as an observer who is observing, you also gain perspective on what you're experiencing. As you gain perspective, you develop your ability to not fuse with what you're experiencing. Then, you're more able to respond to situations and circumstances with actions that are in alignment with the reality of what you're observing. As your capacity to be an observer who is not caught up in what you're observing grows, so does your capacity for experiencing self-kindness, self-compassion, inner peace, joy, and well-being.

Phase 3

During the third phase, your attention shifts to understanding that your sense of being a separate self, separate observer, or separate "I" is not stable or steady. In fact, like your sensations, emotions, and thoughts, your sense of being a separate self is a changing experience. Your felt-sense of being a unique and separate observer comes and goes. Sometimes it's present. Sometimes it's absent. When your sense of self is absent, you're simply *being*. As you grow your capacity to simply *be*, you're growing your capacity to understand that your belief in being a separate self or "I" is not the whole story. You're more than a separate self. You're more than all the personal movements of your body, senses, and mind. Your sense of self and all of your personal movements arise and pass away *in* awareness.

During this third phase of iRest, you begin to feel yourself *as* unchanging awareness. As unchanging awareness, you experience how all the changing movements of your body, mind, senses, and even your felt-sense of being—and being a separate self—arise and pass away in awareness.

Phase 4

During the fourth phase, your attention turns to experiencing yourself *as* awareness. Here, you come to understand that there's a difference between *being* and *awareness*. What's the difference? Being is a felt-sense of presence that you're aware *of*. Being is a movement that arises *in* your awareness. During this phase, you recognize how every changing movement, including being, arises and disappears *in* your awareness. During this fourth phase, your attention turns away from every changing object, including the felt-sense of being, and turns to asking the question, "What *is* awareness?"

As your attention focuses on the question "What *is* awareness?" you begin to realize that you can't look at awareness in the same way you would look at an object. Awareness isn't an object. Awareness is arising *in* awareness. Awareness arises in itself. Therefore, to know awareness you have to let go of being an observer of awareness and dissolve into *being awareness*.

During this fourth phase, then, your sense of being a separate observer dissolves into *being awareness*. You become completely absorbed in *being* awareness. Your attention turns away from all changing experiences and into being awareness. Here, you find yourself entering an entirely new dimension of experience.

Phase 5

During the fifth phase, you move beyond any last traces of self-awareness. By self-awareness, I mean the subtle sense of being an observer who is aware of your being awareness. In this fifth phase, all sense of self-awareness dissolves completely into simply *being awareness*. Here, you're no longer aware of being awareness. All sense of self-awareness has gone away.

As self-awareness dissolves, you move into a dimension where "*you* are not." By this, I mean that you move into a dimension of existence where you have no sense of awareness, being, self, "I," or anything else. This dimension is similar to when you're in deep sleep, or when you're driving across an expanse of highway and are without any thoughts, dream images, or sense of self. In this phase of iRest you *are*, but you aren't aware that you are! Then, as self-awareness returns, the "perfume" of where you just were

The iRest Program for Healing PTSD

comes back along with self-awareness. In iRest Yoga Nidra, this "perfume" is called your *essential nature.*

What you are as your essential nature is beyond description and words. Your essential nature is the mystery from which all of life emerges. You are the mystery that is the essence of well-being, health, and wholeness. Your essential nature can never be disturbed by any difficulty, strife, or struggle that you experience during your lifetime. Your essential nature has never been disturbed by trauma or your symptoms of PTSD. Your essential nature is indestructible. It's not capable of being harmed. Experiencing your indestructible wholeness enables you to face your darkest fears and worst nightmares. It allows you to heal and move beyond any and all symptoms of PTSD. Here's one Vietnam vet's account of experiencing the mystery for himself:

> *I wish I'd been taught iRest when I first experienced PTSD. iRest provides the piece that's been missing from all the other PTSD programs I've tried. For the first time since returning from Vietnam, I feel like I have the tools to help me face my worst nightmares. I never wanted to face them before, because I didn't know what to do with them. iRest helps me remember who I really am. The more I practice, the more I see that my life changes for the better. I truly believe that iRest saves my life every day. iRest has given me the hope and strength I needed to reconnect to myself and to the world again. It's the one practice to heal my PTSD that I know I'm going to keep doing.*

Phase 6

During phase 6, you move through your everyday life with a new sense of who you really are. You live your life from your felt-sense of your essential nature, or wholeness. Now, no matter what else you're experiencing, you live your life with the felt-sense of what's always whole and healthy within you. As you embrace your wholeness, self-judgment, helplessness, and hopelessness fall away. When you know who you really are beneath your symptoms of PTSD, hope and energy arrive. Hope and energy enable you to apply the practice and tools of iRest with enthusiasm. Working with the tools of iRest enables you to recognize your anxiety, depression, self-judgment, and hopelessness—all your sensations, emotions, and thoughts—as simply messengers. Once you've responded to these messengers, they no longer need to hang around. Their job is done. With the job done, they simply dissolve into thin air. As these messengers leave, they're replaced with well-being, peace, joy, and the ever-present felt-sense of your underlying wholeness.

Practice 35: Experiencing Your Wholeness

Sit or lie down in a comfortable position. With your eyes open or gently closed, allow your senses to open to the sounds around you...the touch of air on your skin...the sensations where your body touches the surface that it's resting on...and the feeling of letting go into being at rest and at ease throughout your entire body and mind....

Bring attention to sensations in your jaw...mouth...eyes...forehead... neck...shoulders...arms...palms...chest...belly...upper and lower back... pelvis...hips...legs...feet.... Welcome your entire body as a field of radiant sensation...front and back...left and right...inside and out.... Welcome your entire body as a field of radiant sensation....

Be aware of the various movements of sensations, emotions, and thoughts that are coming and going in your awareness.... Take time to relate to them as messengers and see the actions they're asking you to take in your everyday life....

Noting the Observer

Now, turn your attention to sensing yourself as the one who is aware of these changing movements.... Note how you're the observer, the one who is observing.... Let go of attending to the movements and instead note and feel yourself as the one who is observing them.... Feel yourself as an observer who is observing....

Being

As you feel yourself as an observer who is observing, allow yourself to settle into the feeling of being.... Note how, as being, you feel spacious and open... beyond time...perfect and without need...connected within and without, as being...and complete as you are, as being...relaxing into being...without thinking...just being....

Awareness

Note how you're aware of being...how the feeling of being is in your awareness.... Note how the feeling of being—and the various movements of sensation, thinking, and emotion—are all activities arising in your awareness....

Allow your attention to turn away from being toward sensing awareness.... Allow yourself to become absorbed in sensing and being awareness...no thinking...just being awareness....

Notice how awareness is, whether being or thinking is present or absent... how awareness is, whether emotion or sensation is present or absent...how awareness is, whether anything else is present or absent....

Allow attention to be completely absorbed in being awareness...everything dropping away except for the felt-sense of being awareness....

Self-Awareness

Note, as you're being awareness, how you're aware of being awareness... how the feelings of being a self or "I" who is aware is present...and how this sense of self creates a subtle separation between you, who is aware, and awareness...how your sense of "I" maintains awareness as an object that you're aware of.... Allow attention to become even more absorbed in being awareness, so that all sense of self, "I," self-awareness, and separation drops away....

Wholeness

Feel yourself as awareness that is everywhere...infinitely spacious and open... how inside and outside merge together into the felt-sense of wholeness...no inside or outside...just the wholeness of awareness...just experiencing your undivided wholeness that is aware....

Well-Being

Invite in your inner resource of well-being and the feeling of being secure and at peace.... Affirm these as qualities of awareness and wholeness that you can access at a moment's notice whenever you take time to welcome the felt-sense of awareness and your wholeness....

Completion

Continue resting as the felt-sense of wholeness and awareness...experiencing your wholeness until you feel ready to end this practice of iRest. As you're ready to return to your everyday activities, take a few moments to affirm your intention to continue sensing your felt-sense of wholeness, awareness, and well-being throughout your daily life...while you're walking, talking, working, playing, resting, or sleeping.... Continue to welcome the felt-sense of awareness, wholeness, and well-being as present...accompanying your every experience...remembering you...in every moment....

When you're ready to return to your daily activities, take a few moments to open and close your eyes several times while noticing objects in the environment around you, all the while being awareness.... As you begin to move, remain with the felt-sense of being awareness...then go about your day while noticing how the felt-sense of unchanging awareness is always present.

Moving Forward

Knowing yourself as wholeness enables you to experience your essential nature that's incapable of being harmed or injured. Wholeness *is* your essential nature. As such, it's *always* present. Even when you forget your wholeness, it's always waiting within you to be remembered. As you move forward, continually make it your intention to remember and experience your wholeness throughout your daily activities. Affirm this intention and one day you'll realize how your wholeness has been, and is always, with you. It's your ultimate inner resource. It's your friend for life. It's an ally who's always here to support you to realize and experience your basic health and well-being, in every moment.

Chapter 12

Bringing It All Together

iRest gives me a break from life, gives me peace, and helps me remember who I am inside. The more I do the practice, the more I see my life change for the better. I truly believe that iRest saves me—every day. iRest gives me the hope and strength I need to reconnect with myself and the world again.

—US Marine, after three tours
of duty

iRest is a program that helps you heal your PTSD. The iRest program is also a way to live your life. I believe this because the program teaches you how to respond to every moment in your life, wherever you are, whatever you're doing, whomever you're with. Based on my knowledge of, experience with, and belief in the iRest program, I invite you, as I have, to make iRest your practice for life. The tools of iRest can easily be adapted to your day-to-day needs, so that you can use them 24 hours a day, 7 days a week, 365 days a year—for the rest of your life.

You can practice each iRest tool one after the other, or you can jump from tool to tool, skipping the ones that don't meet your needs in the moment. How you use the iRest program in your daily life depends, quite simply, on you and your needs in each moment. What's most important is that you create the practice that's right for you, knowing that as your needs change over time, so will your practice of iRest.

In this chapter, I focus on how to use all ten tools together as the complete iRest Program for Healing PTSD. This chapter also continues to focus on the iRest program as a way of living your life so that you feel in harmony with yourself, your relationships, and with life itself in every moment of your life, no matter your circumstance.

As with each individual tool, the complete practice of iRest is organized around the core principle of welcoming. In this chapter I'll first review this core principle of welcoming, and then show you the complete practice of iRest.

Welcoming: Your Perfect Response to Each Moment

Welcoming is the core principle of the iRest program. It underlies each tool, as well as the complete iRest practice.

Embracing the attitude of welcoming helps you meet everything that life brings to you. Welcoming enables you to see how every situation arrives paired with its perfect response. And that perfect response always lies within you!

Welcoming allows you to take a step back from what you're experiencing. Taking a step back permits you to experience yourself first as an observer, then as awareness. Being awareness enables you to realize that you're more than what you're experiencing. Living your life from an attitude of welcoming and being awareness allows you to experience yourself as a unique and creative expression of life. In turn, this enables you to feel yourself in harmony with the wholeness of life, even when disharmony is what's showing up.

To Live in Harmony, Embrace Disharmony

Disharmony is a part of life. Disharmony is also a messenger that asks you to take actions that enable you to restore and maintain harmony in your body and mind.

When a virus infects your body, you get a fever. While in the moment you may feel a sense of disharmony, fever is your body's natural way of fending off a viral infection. Similarly, when you experience trauma, your body manifests symptoms of post-traumatic stress. While these symptoms may make you feel out of harmony with yourself and the world around you, they are your body's natural way of getting your attention; by attending to them, you can restore your felt-sense of harmony and well-being.

Disharmony is simply a natural messenger that's calling you back home to harmony. When disharmony comes, don't turn away from it. Don't try to get rid of it. Resisting or refusing disharmony only leads to greater disharmony. Remember, instead, that disharmony is your body's way of getting your attention. Your willingness to welcome and respond to disharmony, as an ongoing fact of life, enables you to welcome and respond to what life is asking of you in each moment. Doing this supports you to live in harmony with your body, mind, and the world.

Welcome Every Messenger

You know when you're not welcoming the moment. You know when you're separating from your ground of harmony and wholeness. In each case, you have a gut feeling that something's "off" or "not right," or you feel a sense of "separation" in yourself. These feelings are behind all symptoms of PTSD. They are messengers calling for your attention. These feelings are asking you to welcome them and to see what actions you need to take to establish harmony and wholeness within yourself and your life.

So, welcome the feeling that something's "off." Welcome the feeling that something's "not right." Welcome the feeling of being "separate." Allow these feelings to show you the right actions to take in this and every moment. Be willing to welcome and respond to any and all of the messengers that call for your attention. The practice of welcoming the "what is" of each moment supports you to find true health, harmony, and wholeness within yourself.

Remember, every situation always arrives paired with its perfect and appropriate response. The practice of iRest teaches you to recognize and affirm this truth. It provides you with the tools to locate your perfect response so that you can find the actions you need to take to experience healing, health, harmony, and balance in your life.

The Complete Practice of iRest

While each iRest tool can be used on its own, when used together the ten
tools of iRest form a unified, complete practice. When practiced together,
each tool naturally leads to the next tool. For instance, affirming your
heartfelt mission, intention, and inner resource lays the foundation for
experiencing your body as sensation—bodysensing. In turn, bodysensing
lays the foundation for experiencing your body as energy—breathsensing.
Welcoming the messengers of sensation and energy lays the foundation for
experiencing the messengers of emotion and thought. Welcoming messengers of emotion and thought allows you to recognize the actions you
need to take to stay in harmony with yourself and the world around you.
Welcoming these messengers also paves the way for you to experience joy,
well-being, and yourself as the observer of all that you're experiencing.
Taking the stance of an observer enables you to gain perspective, allows
you to feel yourself as being. Experiencing yourself as being permits you to
realize yourself as awareness. Knowing yourself as awareness enables you
to feel your underlying, non-separate wholeness with all of life. Knowing
your wholeness with life allows you to realize and live your heartfelt mission
in your daily life. Each iRest tool supports every other iRest tool to form a
unified circle and complete practice for healing PTSD (see figure 1).

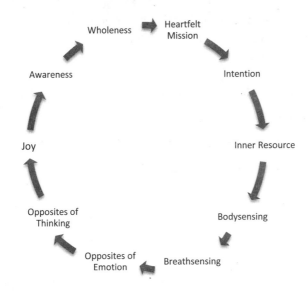

Figure 1. The Unified Circle of iRest

In keeping with this understanding, when you work with the complete practice of iRest, take time to linger with each tool. It takes time for each tool to reveal to you the particular understanding and action that you need to take. Sometimes you'll instantly discover what you need to know and do. At other times, it can take minutes, hours, days, weeks, or even months of practice to come to the right understanding and right action. Remember, healing PTSD is a journey. It's a process that unfolds over time. Be gentle with yourself. Call on patience, persistence, and perseverance to support your daily practice and routines. You're in good company. Millions have walked this path of healing their PTSD before you. They did it. So can you.

What follows are three versions of the complete practice of iRest—as 8-minute, 20-minute, and 35-minute versions. The practice of iRest can take as few as several seconds when you're working with one tool. Or it can take as long as you need when you're working with several or all ten tools together. The important point I want to emphasize is to take as long as you need. My heartfelt desire is for you to make the practice your own, so that iRest becomes an essential practice in your life, for life.

Practice 36: 8-Minute iRest

With your eyes open or closed, welcome the environment and sounds around you...the touch of air on your skin...the sensations where your body touches the surface that's supporting it....

Affirming Your Heartfelt Mission, Intention, and Inner Resource

Welcome and affirm your heartfelt mission...the feeling of life living you with purpose, meaning, and value....

Welcome and affirm your intention...your intention that supports you in realizing your heartfelt mission in your daily life....

Welcome and affirm your inner resource...the felt-sense of well-being... and of being secure and at ease in this and every moment....

Practicing Bodysensing

Bring attention to sensations in your jaw...mouth...ears...eyes...forehead... scalp...neck...shoulders...arms...palms and fingers...torso...legs...feet... your entire body...your body as a field of radiant sensation....

Feel yourself as the observer of all the sensations that are present.... Affirm to yourself, *I am aware...I am at ease...I am safe and secure with myself.*...

Practicing Breathsensing

Sense your body breathing itself...abdomen expanding with each inhalation...abdomen releasing with each exhalation.... With each exhalation, affirm to yourself, *I am aware and at ease...I am aware and at ease.*...

Welcoming Emotions and Thoughts

Note and welcome emotions and thoughts that are present, without trying to change anything...welcoming your experience just as it is.... If it's helpful, note and experience opposites of the emotions and thoughts that are present, all the while noting actions that these messengers are inviting you to take in your life.... Affirm to yourself, *I have within me the perfect response to each moment.*...

Welcoming Joy and Well-Being

Welcome the ease and joy of simply being....

Being an Observer

Welcome yourself as the observer of everything that you're experiencing....

Being Awareness

Note how everything is arising and passing away in your awareness.... Welcome yourself as the spacious openness of awareness...undeniable... indescribable...everywhere...inside...outside....

Experience Your Non-Separate Wholeness

Welcome the feeling of wholeness...yourself as a unique expression of the wholeness of life...while also feeling yourself and everything interconnected and not separate...feeling yourself as a unique expression of the wholeness of life....

Back into Life

As you're ready, open and close your eyes several times while welcoming your inner resource of well-being...feeling grounded and connected to yourself and the world around you...and the feeling of life living you, giving your life a sense of purpose, meaning, and value....

As you're ready, come back to your wide-awake state of mind and body... allowing the feeling of well-being to remain with you as you move back now, into your daily life...feeling gratitude for taking this time for experiencing your health, healing, and wholeness, and for taking this time to practice iRest.

With practice, you can learn to adapt iRest to the time that you have available—one minute, eight minutes, twenty minutes, or longer. With this in mind, you always have the time to practice iRest. Here is an example of a slightly longer practice.

📻 🔊 Practice 37: 20-Minute iRest

With your eyes open or closed, welcome the environment and sounds around you...sensations of warmth or coolness on your skin...the touch of air on your skin...the sensations where your body touches the surface that's supporting it....

Affirm to yourself, *I am aware...I am awake...I am at ease...I am practicing iRest....*

Affirming Your Heartfelt Mission

Welcome your heartfelt mission...the feeling of life living you with purpose, meaning, and value...as you silently affirm to yourself, *I am a unique and valued expression of life.... Life is living me with purpose and meaning....* Experience this as true with your entire body and mind....

Affirming Your Intention

Welcome and affirm your intention...the intention that supports you to realize your heartfelt mission in your daily life...feeling and affirming your intention with your entire body and mind as true in this moment....

Affirming Your Inner Resource

Welcome and affirm your inner resource...the felt-sense of well-being...and of being secure and at ease in this and every moment...the safe haven within you, where you can return whenever you need to take time out to rest, restore, and feel secure and at ease....

Practicing Bodysensing

Welcome sensations that are present throughout your body...starting in your jaw...mouth...ears...the sensation of the breath coming and going at the entrance of your nostrils...the sensation of your eyes....

Sense without going into thinking...the sensation of your forehead... scalp...back of the head and neck....

Sense your left shoulder...left arm...left palm and fingers...right shoulder...right arm...right palm and fingers...both hands, arms, and shoulders at the same time...as radiant sensation....

Sense the entire torso...front and back.... Let go of thinking...just sensing...the entire torso...inside...and outside...as sensation....

Sense your left hip...left leg...left foot...the entire left foot and leg...right hip...right leg...right foot...the entire right foot and leg...both legs together... both legs as sensation....

Sense the entire body...inside...and outside...a field of radiant sensation....

Feel yourself as the observer of all the sensations that are present in your awareness.... Feel yourself just being...aware and awake as the observer of all these sensations....

Affirm to yourself, *I am aware...awake...and resting at ease....*

Practicing Breathsensing

Sense your body breathing.... Welcome the flow of air in the nostrils... throat...the gentle expanding and releasing of the chest and abdomen with each inhalation and exhalation....

Sense your abdomen expanding with each inhalation...abdomen releasing with each exhalation.... With each breath, affirm to yourself, *I am aware and at ease...I am aware and at ease....*

Remain with the feeling of deep release with each exhalation...aware and attentive.... Welcome your inner resource of ease and well-being with each exhalation and inhalation...feeling ease and well-being throughout the entire body....

Feel yourself as the observer of all that's now present in your awareness....

Affirm to yourself, *I am aware...awake...and resting at ease....*

Welcoming Opposites of Feeling and Emotion

Welcome feelings of warmth...ease...and comfort....

And, if present, welcome their opposites.... If you're sensing warmth, welcome coolness...if ease, welcome tension...if comfort, welcome discomfort...without thinking...just sensing and feeling...moving back and forth between opposites at your own pace.... Then, feel both opposites at the same time...while also experiencing how this impacts your body and mind....

Feel yourself as the observer of all the feelings that are present in your awareness....

Welcome an emotion that may be present...or an emotion that you're working with in your life.... If no emotion is present, this, too, is perfect.... Welcome what most calls your attention in this moment.... Feel free to return to your inner resource at any time you wish to take a momentary time-out... to feel secure and at ease....

And if an emotion is present, where and how in your body do you feel it?... Are there thoughts or images that come along with this emotion?... Welcome your experience just as it is, without judging what's present...welcoming it just as it is.... And if it is helpful, locate an opposite of this emotion and where and how you feel it in your body.... Then, move between these opposites...back and forth...at your own pace.... Then, as you're ready, experience both opposites of emotion at the same time, while sensing how this impacts your body and mind....

Feel yourself as the observer of all that's now present in your awareness...just being...aware and awake as the observer of all that's present... affirming to yourself, *I am aware...awake...and resting at ease....*

Welcoming Opposites of Thought

Now, locate a thought or belief that's present...perhaps a belief that you take to be true about yourself.... And, if no belief is present, welcome whatever most calls for your attention.... And, if a thought or belief is present, welcome it as a messenger.... Where and how do you feel this thought or belief in your body when you take it to be true?...

And, if it's helpful, bring to mind the opposite of this belief.... Where and how do you feel this opposite belief in your body when you take it to be true?... Welcome and stay with your experience just as it is....

Then, welcome both beliefs and experience how this impacts your body and mind....

Feel yourself as the observer of all that's now present in your awareness...just being...aware and awake as the observer of all that is present.... Affirm to yourself, *I am aware...awake...and resting at ease....*

Welcoming Joy and Well-Being

Bring attention to sensations of well-being and joy...well-being and joy expanding throughout your entire body...every cell in your body welcoming joy and well-being....

And be aware of all that's now in awareness...while dissolving into being spacious openness in which all these changing activities are coming and going....

Being Awareness

Settle into just being...nothing to do...nowhere to be...just being.... Notice how everything is arising in your awareness.... Feel into being awareness.... Welcome yourself as the space and openness of awareness...undeniable...indescribable...everywhere...in   front...behind...left...right...inside...outside... awareness everywhere....

Experiencing Your Non-Separate Wholeness

Welcome the feeling of the wholeness of life...life living you as one of its unique and perfect expressions...everything interconnected through the underlying essence of life...feeling your wholeness while reflecting upon the different movements that are now present...sensations...emotions... thoughts...well-being...the feeling of being, and being awareness...welcoming everything just as it is....

Back into Life

As you're ready, open and close your eyes several times while welcoming your inner resource of well-being...feeling grounded and connected to yourself and the world around you...and the feeling of life living you...giving your life a sense of purpose, meaning, and value....

Sense the environment around you.... Imagine going about your life affirming to yourself, *I am aware...awake...and at ease in every moment.... I contain within me the perfect response to each and every moment that gives me the felt-sense of health, harmony, and wholeness with myself and all of life.*

When you're ready, come fully back to your wide-awake state...grateful for taking this time for yourself, for health, healing, and experiencing your wholeness, and the practice of iRest.

Feel free to combine or edit any of the scripts in this book, including the ones presented in this chapter. Each script is a learning vehicle. Each is designed to help you make iRest a part of your daily life. What's most important is to not feel hurried when practicing. Adapt the practice to you, not yourself to the practice. When you have time and space, do take up the following 35-minute practice that weaves together all ten tools of iRest.

Practice 38: 35-Minute iRest

Begin your practice of iRest by adjusting your body so that you feel completely supported by the surface you're resting on.... Release unnecessary tension in your jaw...shoulders...arms...torso...legs...your entire body and mind settling into feeling at rest and at ease....

During iRest, welcome every experience you have as a messenger that's here to help you experience health, healing, and well-being at all levels of your body, mind, and spirit.... Welcome every messenger as it arrives with curiosity and openness....

Allow your senses to be open to your environment and the sounds around you.... Welcome the feeling of air touching your skin...the sensations where your body touches the surface that's supporting it...and the feeling of letting go and being at ease throughout your entire body and mind....

Affirming Your Heartfelt Mission

Welcome your heartfelt mission...the feeling of life living you with purpose, meaning, and value...as you silently affirm to yourself, *I am a unique and valued expression of life...life living me with purpose and meaning.*... Experience this as true with your entire body and mind....

Affirming Your Intention

Bring to mind your intention for today's practice...your intention that supports you to live your heartfelt mission...perhaps to remain awake and attentive... or to explore a particular sensation, emotion, or belief.... Feel and affirm your intention with your entire body and mind as true in this moment....

Affirming Your Inner Resource

Bring attention to your inner resource...the place within your body where you experience a felt-sense of well-being...and of being secure and at ease.... If it's helpful, imagine a place, person, or experience that supports you to feel secure and at ease...using all of your senses to enhance your experience.... Imagine sounds, sights, sensations, smells, and tastes that invite ease and well-being into your entire body and mind.... Affirm that you can return to your inner resource at any time, day or night, or during your practice of iRest...whenever you feel the need to take a momentary time-out to rest...to restore...and to feel totally secure and at ease....

Practicing Bodysensing

Rotate your attention through your body while experiencing and welcoming sensations.... You may feel something, or little at all.... Whatever you experience is perfect just as it is....

Sense your jaw...mouth...teeth...lips and gums...tongue...the entire inside of your mouth...the entire jaw and mouth...as sensation.... Give up thinking and simply welcome sensation in the jaw and mouth....

Sense your left ear...right ear...welcoming both ears at the same time as sensation....

Sense your left nostril...right nostril...the flow of air and sensation inside both nostrils.....

Feel the sensation of the left eye...eyebrow...temple...cheekbone...the entire left eye...right eye...eyebrow...temple...cheekbone...the entire right eye.... Welcome both eyes at the same time...as sensation....

Without thinking, just feeling...the sensation of the forehead...scalp...back of the head...neck...the entire face...head...and neck as sensation....

Sense your left shoulder...left upper arm...forearm...wrist...palm and fingers...the sensation of the entire left arm and hand...right shoulder...right upper arm...forearm...wrist...palm and fingers...the sensation of the entire right arm and hand...welcoming both arms and hands at the same time as radiant sensation....

Sense the upper chest...midchest...belly...the sensation of the upper back...midback...lower back...the entire back of the torso...entire front of the torso...the entire torso, front and back...inside and outside...as shimmering sensation....

Bring attention into the pelvis...left hip...left upper leg...knee...lower leg...ankle...and foot...the sensation of the entire left foot...leg...and hip....

Be awake...attentive...yet relaxed and at ease...sensing the right hip...right upper leg...knee...lower leg...ankle...and foot...the sensation of the entire right foot...leg...and hip....

Welcome both hips...legs...and feet...all together as radiant sensation....

Welcome the entire front of the body...a field of sensation...back of the body...left side of the body...right side...inside the body...outside of the body...the entire body as shimmering sensation....

Note how you're the observer...watching all of these sensations coming and going...everything just as it is.... Feel yourself being nonjudging awareness, in which all of these sensations are coming and going....

Silently affirm to yourself, *I'm practicing iRest.... My body is deeply at rest...perhaps even asleep...but I am aware...at ease...attentive and awake....*

Practicing Breathsensing

Sense the body breathing itself and the natural flow of sensation as breath enters and leaves the nostrils...the gentle rise and fall of the abdomen and chest....

Now, begin counting from 1 to 11 while sensing your belly expanding and releasing with each breath, like this: Inhaling, belly expanding, 1; exhaling, belly releasing, 1...inhaling, belly expanding, 2; exhaling, belly releasing, 2; and so on.... With each count, tension releasing throughout your entire body.... Continue counting on your own.... During each exhalation, feel a deep release of tension throughout your body.... With each inhalation, simply remain with the feeling of deep release.... Sensing and releasing tension...welcoming deep relaxation throughout your body.... Awake and attentive.... When you come to 11, or if you happen to lose count, begin again at 1...long, smooth exhalation...tension releasing throughout the entire body...jaw...ears...eyes...forehead...scalp...shoulders...belly... legs.... Tension releasing throughout the whole body...awake...attentive... body breathing itself....

Now, allow the counting to fall away.... Remain attentive to the flows of sensation throughout the body...sensing the body as a field of shimmering sensation....

Sense how you are the observer of all that's now present in your awareness...awake...and aware...of all that's present...sensations...thoughts... images.... Affirm to yourself, *I am aware...awake...practicing iRest...and resting at ease....*

Welcoming Opposites of Feeling and Emotion

Welcome feelings that are present...perhaps the feeling of warmth...heaviness...or the feeling of being at ease...without changing anything, simply welcoming feelings that are present just as they are....

Now, locate opposite feelings.... If you're sensing warmth, find coolness...if heaviness, sense lightness...if ease, then tension...without going into thinking...just sensing.... Then, come back to the original feeling...then, feel its opposite again.... When you're ready, move back and forth between opposites at your own pace....

When it feels right, welcome both opposites at the same time...experiencing how this impacts your entire body and mind...not with thinking...just sensing...just experiencing....

Feel yourself as the observer who's observing all these feelings that are coming and going in your awareness.... Feel yourself being nonjudging awareness, in which all of these movements are coming and going....

Now, welcome an emotion that's present in your body...or recall an emotion that you're working with in your life.... If no emotion is present, be with what's most calling your attention right now...whether an emotion or another sensation....

And remember, you can always return to the safe haven of your inner resource whenever you feel the need to take a momentary time-out to feel secure and at ease....

And if an emotion is present, where and how do you feel it in your body?... Are there thoughts or images that accompany this emotion?... Welcome your experience just as it is without judging or trying to change it....

Now, locate an opposite emotion and where and how you experience this opposite in your body.... If it's helpful, recall a memory that invites this opposite of emotion more fully into your body....

When it feels right, move back and forth between these opposites, experiencing first one, then its opposite, in your own time.... Sense how each emotion affects your body and mind....

Then, sense both emotions at the same time...experiencing how this affects your entire body and mind....

Sense how you are the observer of all that's now present in your awareness...awake...and...aware...of all that's present...sensations...thoughts...images.... Affirm to yourself, *I am aware...and awake...practicing iRest...and resting at ease....*

Welcoming Opposites of Thought

Notice and welcome the various thoughts that are present...thoughts as objects that are coming and going...observing and noting them as they appear and disappear...without getting involved....

If it feels right, welcome a particular group of thoughts that form a belief or self-judgment that you take to be true about yourself and fall into believing at times.... And if no belief is present, this, too, is your experience.... Welcome whatever is most present in this moment....

And if a belief is present, where and how do you feel it in your body when you take it to be true?... Welcome memories, emotions, and sensations that naturally arise without judging or trying to change your experience....

And if this belief had an opposite, what might its opposite be?... Bring to mind the opposite of your belief or self-judgment.... Where and how do you feel it in your body when you take this opposite belief to be true?... There's no right or wrong answer...your experience is perfect just as it is.... Stay with your experience just as it is....

Now, return to the original belief or judgment...welcoming your experience with curiosity and openness.... At your own pace, go back and forth several times between these opposites, experiencing first one, then the other, with your entire body and mind.... When it feels right, welcome both beliefs at the same time...experiencing how this impacts your entire body and mind....

And be aware of all that's now in your awareness...sensing how you are the witness of all that's arising...awake...and aware...of sensations...emotions...thoughts.... Affirm to yourself, *I am aware...and awake...practicing iRest...and resting at ease....*

Welcoming Joy and Well-Being

Bring attention to sensations of well-being or joy in your body...or recall a memory of a particular person, animal, place, or circumstance that invites joy or well-being into your body....

Experience the feeling of well-being or joy expanding throughout your entire body...every cell in your body welcoming its natural sense of joy and well-being.... Perhaps experience an inner smile coming from your heart... throughout your entire body...your lips gently smiling...joy, well-being, and an inner smile flowing throughout your body...face...torso...arms...and legs...your entire body alive with the feeling of well-being and joy....

And be aware of all that's now in awareness, while dissolving into the spacious openness in which all these changing activities are coming and going....

And be aware of all that's now in your awareness...sensing how you're the observer of all that's arising...awake...and aware of sensations...emotions...thoughts...joy.... Affirm to yourself, *I am aware...and awake...practicing iRest...and resting at ease....*

Being Awareness

Now, set aside thinking and memory and settle into simply being...nothing to do...nowhere to be...just the delightful feeling of being....

Notice how you're aware of being an observer of this feeling of being and everything that you're experiencing.... Allow yourself to dissolve into "being observing"..."being awareness"...all sense of separation dissolving.... Be awareness, in which everything is arising.... Sense how all your thoughts, emotions, sensations, and sounds are simply movements in awareness.... Feel yourself as the spacious openness of awareness...how, as awareness, you're everywhere...nowhere specific...yet undeniably present...as awareness...in front...behind...left...right...inside...outside...formless...yet undeniably present....

Rest here being awareness...feeling your non-separate wholeness with all of life...awake...aware...at ease...everything just as it is...sensing your non-separate wholeness...connected to yourself...the world around you... and all of life.... Reside here being until you're naturally called to end this practice of iRest.

Back into Life

As you're ready to return to your eyes-open state, take a few moments and welcome the feeling of gratitude for taking this time to experience your wholeness, health, and healing...and for taking time for practicing iRest.... Know that as you return to your daily life and activities, you are the underlying, non-separate wholeness of life...seemingly separate but, in fact, never separate... always whole and not separate from all of life....

As you're ready, open and close your eyes several times while feeling your wholeness and welcoming your inner resource of well-being....

Welcome and affirm again your heartfelt mission with your entire body... the sense of life living you with meaning, purpose, and value....

Affirm your intentions that support you living your heartfelt mission....

Affirm the truth that, in every moment, you always have within you the perfect response to each situation and circumstance in your life....

Feel again your body...senses open to the environment and sounds around you.... Imagine going about your day...all the while awake and aware as your undivided wholeness in which all of life is unfolding....

Take your time now...transitioning back into your everyday waking life at your own pace...your body fully awakening to its natural state of eyes open... awakening to its wakeful presence...attentive...awake...aware of your surroundings.... Come fully back when you're ready...grateful for taking this time for yourself...for the practice of iRest...for health...healing...and experiencing your wholeness with all of life.

Additional Meditations

Make the practice of iRest your own! To stay inspired, creative, and playful in your practice, feel free to weave in music, drawing, painting, collage, journaling, and other experiences that draw upon your five senses. For example, I sometimes play music at the end of an iRest practice. I note how the sound affects my body and mind, and supports my ability to welcome the different emotions and images that the music evokes. After an iRest practice, I sometimes take out paper and colored pencils and draw images that best represent the emotions, beliefs, or images I experienced during my practice. I also take time to write down my reflections regarding my experiences during the practice.

Each of these additions to the practice is a way to enhance, support, and deepen your practice of welcoming. Linking forms of artistic expression with your iRest practice can help you recognize more clearly the messengers who arrive during your practice. In turn, you'll be better able to understand the actions you need to take. With understanding and clarity in place, you can easily take these actions back into your daily activities. Follow your creative impulses. Discover ways of energizing your practice so that you look forward to working with iRest throughout your daily life.

My heartfelt desire and intention is that this book inspires you to take up the iRest program as a means to examine every aspect of your life—your relationships, work, creativity, exercise, diet, lifestyle choices, et cetera—and come to understand how the basic principles of iRest support you.

Just so, I'd like to share with you two more practices that you can weave into your practice of iRest. These practices support your healing process, as well as your life in general.

Gratitude. Right Here. Right Now. For No Reason at All.

Gratitude can arise as a warm feeling you have when you feel thankful or appreciative, or when you feel kindness toward yourself or another. It can be a warm feeling of thankfulness that you feel for being alive, or a warm feeling you feel for no reason at all. You just find yourself feeling grateful. Gratitude for no reason at all! This is what happens the more you practice iRest.

Gratitude—like love, peace, and joy—manifests the more you practice iRest. Feeling gratitude for no reason at all happens the more you experience your undivided wholeness. The more you practice iRest, and the more you experience your wholeness, the more gratitude you feel. The more you experience gratitude, the easier it becomes to access, feel, and express gratitude. Take time, then, to experience *gratitude moments* each and every day. For instance, take time each night to note what you're grateful for before falling asleep. (See Day's Review, below.) Or take time each morning and throughout each day to feel gratitude, for no reason at all. You'll find that you feel happier as you move through your day.

▣ ◈ Practice 39: The Practice of Gratitude

With your eyes open or closed, welcome the environment and sounds around you…sensations of warmth or coolness on your skin…the touch of air on your skin…the sensations where your body touches the surface that's supporting it.…

Bring your attention to yourself or to another toward whom you feel, or would like to feel, gratitude.… Think of what you or the other person has said or done for which you feel gratitude.… Notice the sensations, emotions, and thoughts that come to you as you think of yourself or this person and what you, she, or he did or said.… In your imagination, tell yourself or this person how grateful or thankful you feel toward yourself, him, or her.… As you say these words, imagine and notice how you or the other person responds. Notice how these words and the feeling of gratitude affect your body, mind, emotions, and thoughts.…

Imagine writing a letter to yourself or to this person that you might send or just keep to yourself. Or imagine expressing your gratitude directly to yourself or to the other in person.

Be aware of how you feel as you write the letter or communicate in person.… Be aware of the sensations, emotions, and thoughts that you experience as you express your gratitude in your imagination, through your written words, or in person.

As you reflect on the feeling of gratitude that you experience toward another or yourself, note where and how this feeling arises in your body and impacts your mind.... At some point, let go of thinking about what you're grateful for and just experience the feeling of gratitude, without attaching the feeling to a person, activity, or action.... Welcome the feeling of gratitude, just as it is...right here...right now...for no reason at all!... Then, as you go about your day, welcome the feeling of gratitude without attaching it to a specific activity or person.... Feel gratitude just for the sake of feeling gratitude.... Feel how this affects your body...mind...and your day.

Every evening, before falling asleep, take time, as I do, to do a *day's review.* After you've said your good-nights and turned off the lights, take a few quiet moments to reflect on your day. When you do this exercise each evening before bed, you will be pleasantly surprised, as I have been, to experience how your life unfolds more easily the following day.

Practice 40: Day's Review

Take a few moments and welcome the environment and sounds around you...the touch of air on your skin...the sensations where your body touches the surface that's supporting it....

Now, search out moments from your day that feel *unfinished.*... Then, imagine redoing each of these unfinished moments. Imagine the ways you would have liked the situations to have unfolded...what you would have liked to have said or done...and what the others involved would then have said or done.... Like watching a movie, replay scenes over and over again until you feel a sense of, *Ah, that feels perfect.... That's the way I would like to have lived that moment....*

Then—not just in your mind's imagination, but with your entire body, heart, and mind, feel the completion of each event as if it had truly happened that way.... Replay each scene again in this new way, feeling that this is the way you lived these moments.... As you replay each scene, take time to weave your inner resource into what you're experiencing.... Take time to nourish feelings of love, gratitude, peace, and joy into your entire body.... Then, carry the sense of completion and the feelings of gratitude, love, joy, and well-being with you into your sleep.

Moving Forward: Final Words

There are many ways to practice iRest. The practices I've included throughout this book—as well as online as downloadable MP3 recordings—are designed to teach you the core principles of iRest and how to weave them into your daily life. My intention in writing this book is to describe and demonstrate the basic principles and practices of iRest so that you can make this practice your own.

Feel free to change the words that I use. Find your own words, ones that feel "right" and comfortable to you. Take time to practice all ten tools together. Take time to practice each tool, one at a time, over and over. Get to know each tool. Allow each tool to become your trusted friend that you can depend and call on in any time of need.

The practice of yoga nidra has been around for thousands of years. It's survived as a powerful practice of healing and awakening because it works. My intention in writing this book is to show you iRest as a modern-day practice of yoga nidra. I want you to experience how this ancient practice respects your age, culture, religion, and philosophical orientation while it enables you to experience healing, health, well-being, and wholeness at all levels of your life—physical, psychological, and spiritual.

Practice iRest regularly. Integrate it into all aspects of your daily life. Allow iRest to work for you. Then, feel free to pass on what you've learned. Pay forward your experience and understanding of this healing practice. Sharing what you've learned is what iRest and the wholeness it connects you to is all about. Let others know how the practice has worked for you. Invite others to take up this wondrous practice of healing, health, and well-being. This is what your journey of healing your PTSD is all about. This is what our journey as human beings is all about.

As you welcome your wholeness, you become a light for those who follow in your footsteps. We are all brothers and sisters on our healing journey together. May you be a light unto yourself, so that those who follow in your footsteps can also affirm, *If he or she can heal his or her PTSD, I can heal my PTSD.*

Practice 41: A Final Meditation

Take a moment as you are, right now, and be aware of sounds in and around you.... Be aware of the sensations, emotions, and thoughts that are present in your body and mind....

Be aware of your body breathing itself....

Welcome the felt-sense of simply being....

Welcome the felt-sense of being awareness....

Welcome the felt-sense of your non-separate wholeness...the feeling of connection with yourself and the world around you....

Remain here, just being your wholeness....

So simple...so necessary....

Now, go into your day with this underlying feeling of being and wholeness that is always with you....

Throughout your day, notice how the feelings of being, awareness, and wholeness naturally arise.... Allow the practice of iRest to become your 24-hours-a-day, 7-days-a-week, 365-days-a-year lifetime adventure.

Resources

The iRest Program for Healing PTSD

Integrative Restoration Institute
For information on the iRest program contact:
Integrative Restoration Institute
900 5th Ave., Suite 204
San Rafael, CA 94901
(415) 456-3909
info@iRest.us
http://www.iRest.us

The iRest for PTSD Audio Practice Series
All of the guided practices in this book can be downloaded as audio recordings from http://www.irest.us/practices

iRest Trainings, Retreats, and Classes
http://www.irest.us/events

Research on iRest Yoga Nidra
http://www.irest.us/research

Post-Traumatic Stress Disorder

National Center for PTSD
http://www.ptsd.va.gov
https://www.facebook.com/VAPTSD

Trauma Center at Justice Resource Institute
http://www.traumacenter.org

National Institute of Mental Health for PTSD
http://www.nimh.nih.gov/health/topics/post-traumatic-stress-disorder-ptsd/index.shtml

National Suicide Prevention Lifeline
To talk to a trained suicide counselor toll-free:
24-hour hotline: (800) 273-TALK (800-273-8255)
TTY: (800) 799-4TTY (800-799-4889)

References

Angelone, A. and N. Coulter. 1964. "Respiratory Sinus Arrhythmia: A Frequency-Dependent Phenomenon." *Journal of Applied Physiology* 19: 479–482.

Bahari, M. 2011. *Then They Came for Me: A Family's Story of Love, Captivity, and Survival.* New York: Random House.

Baraz, J., and S. Alexander. 2010. *Awakening Joy.* New York: Bantam Books.

Baumann, P., and M. Taft. 2011. *Ego: The Fall of the Twin Towers and the Rise of an Enlightened Humanity.* San Francisco: NE Press.

Benson, H. 2000. *The Relaxation Response.* New York: HarperTorch.

Berk, L., and S. A. Tan. 1995. "Eustress of Mirthful Laughter Modulates the Immune System Lymphokine Interferon-Gamma." *Annals of Behavioral Medicine Supplement, Proceedings of the Society of Behavioral Medicine's Sixteenth Annual Scientific Sessions* 17: C064.

Berk, L., S. A. Tan, and W. Fry. 1993. "Eustress of Humor Associated Laughter Modulates Specific Immune System Components." *Annals of Behavioral Medicine Supplement, Proceedings of the Society of Behavioral Medicine's Fourteenth Annual Scientific Sessions* 15: S111.

Berk, L., S. A. Tan, W. F. Fry, B. J. Napier, J. W. Lee, R. W. Hubbard, J. E. Lewis, and W. C. Eby. 1989. "Neuroendocrine and Stress Hormone Changes During Mirthful Laughter." *American Journal of the Medical Sciences* 298 (6): 390–396.

Berk, L., S. A. Tan, B. Napier, and W. Evy. 1989. "Eustress of Mirthful Laughter Modifies Natural Killer Cell Activity." *Clinical Research* 37: 115A.

Berk, L., S. A. Tan, S. Nehlsen-Cannarella, B. J. Napier, J. E. Lewis, J. E. Lee, and W. C. Eby. 1988. "Humor Associated with Laughter Decreases Cortisol and Increases Spontaneous Lymphocyte Blastogenesis." *Clinical Research* 36: 435A.

Bly, R. 2004. *Kabir: Ecstatic Poems.* Boston, MA: Beacon Press.

Boykin, K. 1998. "Meditation Hints from the Colorado Division of Wildlife." *Shambala Sun*, January, Halifax, Nova Scotia.

Breines, J., and S. Chen. 2012. "Self-Compassion Increases Self-Improvement Motivation." *Personality and Social Psychology Bulletin*, May 29.

Bremner, J. 2006. "Traumatic Stress: Effects on the Brain." *Dialogues in Clinical Neuroscience* 8 (4): 445–61.

Briere, J., and C. Scott. 2006. *Principles of Trauma Therapy: A Guide to Symptoms, Evaluation, and Treatment*. Thousand Oaks, CA: Sage Publications.

Carlson, C. R., and R. H. Hoyle. 1993. "Efficacy of Abbreviated Progressive Muscle Relaxation Training: A Quantitative Review of Behavioral Medicine Research." *Journal of Consulting and Clinical Psychology* December 61 (6): 1059–1067.

Carlson, N. 2012. *Physiology of Behavior*. Pearson Education: Canada.

Clarke, J. 1981. "Lung Capacity and Breathing Patterns During Rest, Exercise, and Illness." *Research Bulletin* 3, No. 2.

DCoE. 2010. "PTSD: Treatment Options." Arlington, VA: Defense Centers of Excellence for Psychological Health and Traumatic Brain Injury. http://dcoe .health.mil/ForHealthPros/PTSDTreatmentOptions.aspx.

Dispenza, J. 2012. *Breaking the Habit of Being Yourself: How to Lose Your Mind and Create a New One*. Carlsbad, CA: Hay House.

Eagleman, D. 2011. *Incognito: The Secret Lives of the Brain*. New York: Pantheon Books.

Eckberg, D. L., Y. T. Kifle, and V. L. Roberts. 1980. "Phase Relationship Between Human Respiration and Baroreflex Responsiveness." *Journal of Physiology* (London) 302: 489–502.

Eckholdt, K., K. Bodmann, H. Cammann, B. Pfeifer, E. Schubert, and U. Kesper. 1976. "Sinus Arrhythmia and Heart Rate in Hypertonic Disease." *Advances in Cardiology* 16: 366–369.

Emmons R. A., and M. E. McCullough. 2003. "Counting Blessings Versus Burdens: An Experimental Investigation of Gratitude and Subjective Well-Being in Daily Life." *Journal of Personality and Social Psychology* 84 (2): 377–389.

Engel, C., C. Goertz, D. Cockfield, D. Armstrong, W. Jonas, J. Walter, et al. 2006. *Yoga Nidra as an Adjunctive Therapy for Post-Traumatic Stress Disorder: A Feasibility Study*. Alexandria, VA: Samueli Institute and Department of Defense Deployment Health Clinical Center and Walter Reed Army Medical Center. Uniformed Services University of the Health Sciences: MILCAM 2003: Contract MDA905-03-C-0003.

Foa, E. B., and S. P. Cahill. 2002. "Specialized Treatment for PTSD: Matching Survivors to the Appropriate Modality." In *Treating Trauma Survivors with PTSD*, edited by R. Yehuda, 43–62. Washington, DC: American Psychiatric Publishing.

Fried, I., C. Wilson, K. MacDonald, and E. Behnke. 1998. "Electric Current Stimulates Laughter." *Nature*, February 12 391 (6668): 650.

Fried, R. 1987. *The Hyperventilation Syndrome: Research and Treatment*. Baltimore, MD: Johns Hopkins University Press.

Fried, R. 1990. *The Breath Connection*. New York: Insight/Plenum.

Fried, R., S. Rubin, M. Fox, and R. Carlton. 1983. *Method and Protocols for Assessing Hyperventilation and Its Treatment*. New York: International Center for the Disabled.

Fritts, M., and M. Khusid. 2014. "Self-Care Meditation Approaches Used Adjunctively in PTSD Management." *Changing the Practice and Perception of Psychiatry.* New York: American Psychiatric Association.

Gendlin, E. T. 1982. *Focusing.* New York: Bantam Books.

Gerdes, L. 2008. *Limitless You: The Infinite Possibilities of a Balanced Brain.* Vancouver, Canada: Namaste Publishing.

Gilbert, J. 2007. "A Brief for the Defense." In *Dancing with Joy,* edited by R. Housden. New York: Random House.

Graham, L. 2013. *Bouncing Back: Rewiring Your Brain for Maximum Resilience and Well-Being.* Novato, CA: New World Library.

Grant, A. M., and F. Gino. 2010. "A Little Thanks Goes a Long Way: Explaining Why Gratitude Expressions Motivate Prosocial Behavior." *Journal of Personality and Social Psychology,* 98 (6): 946–955.

Grossman, Paul. 1983. "Respiration, Stress, and Cardiovascular Function." *Psychophysiology* 20, May: 284–300.

Hanson, R. 2009. *Buddha's Brain.* Oakland, CA: New Harbinger Publications.

Hanson, R. 2013. *Hardwiring Happiness.* New York: Harmony Books.

Hebb, D. 1949 (reprinted 2002). *The Organization of Behavior: A Neuropsychological Theory.* Mahwah, NJ: Lawrence Erlbaum Associates, Inc.

Hincle, L. E., S. T. Carver, and A. Plakun. 1972. "Slow Heart Rates and Increased Risk of Cardiac Death." *Archives of Internal Medicine* 129: 732–750.

Hirsch, J. A., and B. Bishop. 1981. "Respiratory Sinus Arrhythmia in Humans: How Breathing Patterns Modulate Heart Rate." *American Journal of Physiology* 241: 620–629.

Hölzel, B. K., J. Carmody, K. C. Evans, E. A. Hoge, J. A. Dusek, L. Morgan, R. K. Pitman, and S. W. Lazar. 2009. "Stress Reduction Correlates with Structural Changes in the Amygdala." *Social Cognitive and Affective Neuroscience,* March 5 (1): 11–17.

Hutcherson, C., E. Seppala, and J. Gross. 2008. "I Don't Know You But I Like You: Loving Kindness Meditation Increases Positivity Toward Others." Paper presentation at the 6th annual conference Integrating Mindfulness-Based Interventions into Medicine, Health Care & Society. Worcester, MA.

Jacobson, E. 1938. *Progressive Relaxation.* Chicago: University of Chicago Press.

Johnston, L. C. 1980. "The Abnormal Heart Rate Response to a Deep Breath in Borderline Labile Hypertension: A Sign of Autonomic Nervous System Dysfunction." *American Heart Journal* 99: 487–493.

Kessler, R. C., P. Berglund, O. Demler, R. Jin, K. R. Merikangas, and E. E. Walters. 2005. "Lifetime Prevalence and Age-of-Onset Distributions of DSM-IV Disorders in the National Comorbidity Survey Replication." *Archives of General Psychiatry,* June, 62 (6): 593–602.

Kleber, R., C. R. Figley, and B. Gersons. 1995. *Beyond Trauma: Cultural and Societal Dynamics.* New York: Plenum Press.

Kosfeld, M., M. Heinrichs, P. Zak, U. Fischbacher, and E. Fehr. 2005. "Oxytocin Increases Trust in Humans." *Nature* 435 (7042): 673–676.

Lambert, N. M., and F. D. Fincham. 2011. "Expressing Gratitude to a Partner Leads to More Relationship Maintenance Behavior." *Emotion* 11 (1): 52–60.

Lemonick, M. 2005. "The Biology of Joy." *Time Magazine.* January 17.

Luthe, W., and J. H. Schultz. 1969. *Autogenic Therapy.* New York: Grune and Stratton.

Lutz, A., J. Brefczynski-Lewis, T. Johnstone, and R. Davidson. 2008. "Regulation of the Neural Circuitry of Emotion by Compassion Meditation: Effects of Meditative Expertise." *PLoS ONE* 3 (3): e1897.

McGonigal, K. 2012. *The Neuroscience of Change: A Compassion-Based Program for Personal Transformation.* Boulder, CO: Sounds True.

Mednick, S., and M. Erhman. 2006. *Take a Nap! Change Your Life.* New York: Workman Publishing Company.

Metzinger, T. 2009. *The Ego Tunnel.* New York: Basic Books.

Miller, R. 1991. "Psychophysiology of Respiration: Western and Eastern Perspectives." *Journal of International Association of Yoga Therapists* II.

Miller, R. 2003. "Welcoming All That Is: Yoga Nidra and the Play of Opposites in Psychotherapy." In *The Sacred Mirror: Nondual Wisdom & Psychotherapy,* edited by J. J. Prendergast, P. Fenner, and S. Krystal. New York: Paragon.

Miller, R. 2005. *Yoga Nidra: A Meditative Practice for Deep Relaxation and Healing.* Boulder, CO: Sounds True.

Miller, R. 2006. "Your Brain on Yoga Nidra: Questions for Richard Miller." *KYTA Bulletin: Winter.* Stockbridge, MA: Kripalu Center for Yoga and Health.

Miller, R. 2013. *Level I Training Manual: Integrative Restoration – iRest.* San Rafael, CA: Integrative Restoration Institute.

Moore, M., D. Brown, N. Money, and M. Bates. 2011. *Mind-Body Skills for Regulating the Autonomic Nervous System.* Arlington, VA: Defense Centers of Excellence for Psychological Health and Traumatic Brain Injury.

Morey, R., A. Gold, K. LaBar, S. Beall, V. Brown, C. Haswell, J. Nasser, R. Wagner, and M. Gregory. 2012. "Amygdala Volume Changes in Posttraumatic Stress Disorder in a Large Case-Controlled Veterans Group." *Archives of General Psychiatry* 69 (11): 1169–1178.

Najavits, L. M. 2007. "Psychosocial Treatments for Posttraumatic Stress Disorder." In *A Guide to Treatments That Work,* edited by P. E. Nathan and J. M. Gorman, 513–530. New York: Oxford University Press.

Novey, D. 2000. *Clinician's Complete Reference to Complementary and Alternative Medicine.* New York: C. V. Mosby, Co.

Pennebaker, J. W., and C. K. Chung. 2007. "Expressive Writing, Emotional Upheavals, and Health." In *Foundations of Health Psychology,* edited by H. Friedman and R. Silver. New York: Oxford University Press.

Pennebaker, J. W. 2001. "Disclosing and Sharing Emotion: Psychological, Social, and Health Consequences." In *Handbook of Bereavement Research: Consequences, Coping, and Care,* edited by M. S. Stroebe, W. Stroebe, R. O. Hansson, and H. Schut, 517–539. Washington, DC: American Psychological Association.

Porges, S. 2001. "The Polyvagal Theory: Phylogenetic Substrates of a Social Nervous System." *International Journal of Psychophysiology* 42: 123–146.

Rama, B. R., and A. Hymes. 1979. *Science of Breath.* Honesdale, PA: Himalayan Press.

Ready, D. J., S. Pollack, R. Olasov, and R. Alarcon. 2006. "Virtual Reality Exposure for Veterans with Posttraumatic Stress Disorder." In *Trauma Treatment Techniques: Innovative Trends,* edited by J. Garrick and M. .B. Williams, 199–200. Binghamton, NY: Haworth Press.

Robotham, D., L. Chakkalackal, and E. Cyhlarova. 2011. *Sleep Matters: The Impact of Sleep on Health and Wellbeing.* London, UK: Mental Health Foundation.

Rodriguez, T. 2013. "Negative Emotions Are Key to Well-Being." *Scientific American Mind* 24: 2.

Roemer, L., and S. M. Orsillo. 2003. "Mindfulness: A Promising Intervention Strategy in Need of Further Study." *Clinical Psychology: Science and Practice* 10 (2): 172–178.

Ross, A., and A. Steptoe. 1980. "Attenuation of the Diving Reflex in Man by Mental Stimulation." *Journal of Physiology* 302: 387–393.

Sansone, R. A., and L. A. Sansone. 2010. "Gratitude and Well Being: The Benefits of Appreciation." *Psychiatry* 7 (11): 18–22.

Saraswati, S. S. 1998. *Yoga Nidra.* New Delhi, India: Bihar School of Yoga.

Schoomaker, E. B. 2010. *Pain Management Task Force: Providing a Standardized DoD and VHA Vision and Approach to Pain Management to Optimize the Care for Warriors and their Families.* Washington, DC: Office of the Army Surgeon General.

Segal, D. 2007. *The Mindful Brain: Reflection and Attunement in the Cultivation of Well-Being.* New York: W. W. Norton.

Seligman, D. 2011. *Flourish.* New York: Free Press.

Seligman, D. 2002. *Authentic Happiness: Using the New Positive Psychology to Realize Your Potential for Lasting Fulfillment.* New York: Free Press.

Seligman, M. E. P., T. A. Steen, N. Park, and C. Peterson. 2005. "Empirical Validation of Interventions." *American Psychologist* 60 (1): 410–421.

Sesana, L. 2013. "The Ancient Greek Theater at Epidaurus." *The Washington Post,* August 23.

Shin, L., S. Rauch, and R. Pitman. 2006. "Amygdala, Medial Prefrontal Cortex, and Hippocampal Function in PTSD." *Annals of the New York Academy of Science* 1071: 67–79.

Stanescu, D., B. Nemery, C. Veriter, and C. Marechal. 1981. "Pattern of Breathing and Ventilatory Response to CO_2 in Subjects Practicing Hatha-Yoga." *Journal of Applied Physiology,* December, (5): 1625–1629.

Stetter, F., and S. Kupper. 2002. "Autogenic Training: A Meta-Analysis of Clinical Outcome Studies." *Applied Psychophysiology and Biofeedback,* March, 27 (1): 45–98.

Tick, E. 2005. *War and the Soul: Healing Our Nation's Veterans from Post-Traumatic Stress Disorder.* Wheaton, IL: Quest Books.

Trzebski, A., M. Raczkowska, and L. Kubin. 1978. "Sinus Arrhythmia and Respiratory Modulation of the Carotid Baroreceptor Reflex in Man." *European Journal of Clinical Investigation* 8: 332.

Van Liempt, S. 2012. "Sleep Disturbances and PTSD: A Perpetual Circle?" *European Journal of Psychotraumatology* 3.

Weathers, F. W., B. T. Litz, J. A. Huska, and T. M. Keane. 1994. *PCL-C Civilian PTSD Checklist.* Washington, DC: National Center for PTSD. Behavioral Science Division. Government document in the public domain. http://mirecc.va.gov/docs/visn6/3_PTSD_CheckList_and_Scoring.pdf and http://www.PDHealth.mil.

Weniger, G., C. Lange, and E. Irle. 2009. "Reduced Amygdala and Hippocampus Size in Trauma-Exposed Women with Borderline Personality Disorder and Without Posttraumatic Stress Disorder." *Journal of Psychiatry & Neuroscience* 34 (5): 383–388.

Williams, L., K. Brown, D. Palmer, B. Liddell, A. Kemp, G. Olivieri, A. Peduto, and E. Gordon. 2006. "The Mellow Years: Neural Basis of Improving Emotional Stability over Age." *Journal of Neuroscience,* June, 26 (24): 6422–6430.

Wilson, J. P., M. J. Friedman, and J. D. Lindy. 2001. *Treating Psychological Trauma and PTSD.* New York: Guilford Press.

Yongue, B. G., S. W. Porges, and P. M. McCabe. 1980. "Changes in Vagal Control of the Heart Following Signaled and Unsignaled Shock." *Psychophysiology* 17: 314.

Zak, P. 2012. *The Moral Molecule.* New York: Dutton Penguin Group.

Richard C. Miller, PhD, is a clinical psychologist, author, researcher, scholar, and meditation teacher. For over forty years, he has devoted his life and work to integrating the teachings of Yoga, Tantra, Advaita, Taoism, and Buddhism with Western psychology. Miller is founding president of the Integrative Restoration Institute and cofounder of the International Association of Yoga Therapists. He was a founding member and past president of the Institute for Spirituality and Psychology, and serves as a senior advisor to the Baumann Foundation.

Foreword writer **Eric B. Schoomaker, MD, PhD**, is a retired US Lieutenant General, as well as former US Army Surgeon General and Commanding General of the US Army Medical Command. He is an internal medicine physician with a PhD in human genetics. While in uniform, he held many assignments, including command of the Walter Reed Army Medical Center in Washington, DC, the Army's Medical Research and Materiel Command at Fort Detrick, MD, an Army academic medical center, a community hospital, deployable medical brigade, and two Army regional medical commands. Schoomaker is the recipient of numerous military awards, including those from France and Germany, the 2012 Dr. Nathan Davis Award from the American Medical Association for outstanding government service, and an Honorary Doctor of Science from Wake Forest University.

Foreword writer **Audrey Schoomaker, RN**, is project coordinator for a research study in therapeutic yoga for the Defense and Veterans Center for Integrative Pain Management. She is an experienced yoga instructor with diverse experience in the field of healing as an Army nurse, nurse educator, and certified mind-body medicine practitioner.

FROM OUR PUBLISHER—

As the publisher at New Harbinger and a clinical psychologist since 1978, I know that emotional problems are best helped with evidence-based therapies. These are the treatments derived from scientific research (randomized controlled trials) that show what works. Whether these treatments are delivered by trained clinicians or found in a self-help book, they are designed to provide you with proven strategies to overcome your problem.

Therapies that aren't evidence-based—whether offered by clinicians or in books—are much less likely to help. In fact, therapies that aren't guided by science may not help you at all. That's why this New Harbinger book is based on scientific evidence that the treatment can relieve emotional pain.

This is important: if this book isn't enough, and you need the help of a skilled therapist, use the following resources to find a clinician trained in the evidence-based protocols appropriate for your problem. And if you need more support—a community that understands what you're going through and can show you ways to cope—resources for that are provided below, as well.

Real help is available for the problems you have been struggling with. The skills you can learn from evidence-based therapies will change your life.

Matthew McKay, PhD
Publisher, New Harbinger Publications

If you need a therapist, the following organization can help you find a therapist trained in cognitive behavioral therapy (CBT).

The Association for Behavioral & Cognitive Therapies (ABCT) Find-a-Therapist service offers a list of therapists schooled in CBT techniques. Therapists listed are licensed professionals who have met the membership requirements of ABCT and who have chosen to appear in the directory.

Please visit www.abct.org and click on *Find a Therapist*.

For additional support for patients, family, and friends, please contact the following:

National Center for PTSD
Visit www.ptsd.va.gov

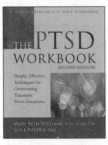
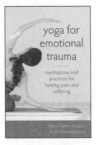
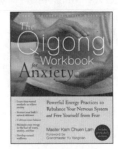
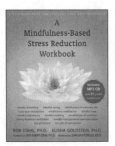
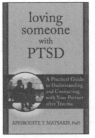
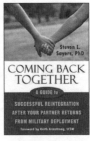